PURKINJE'S VISION

The Dawning of Neuroscience

PURKINJE'S VISION

The Dawning of Neuroscience

by
Nicholas J. Wade and Josef Brožek
in collaboration with Jiří Hoskovec

Routledge
Taylor & Francis Group
NEW YORK AND LONDON

First published by Lawrence Erlbaum Associates, Inc., Publishers
10 Industrial Avenue
Mahwah, NJ 07430

This edition published 2012 by Routledge
711 Third Avenue, New York, NY 10017
2 Park Square, Milton Park, Abingdon, Oxfordshire OX14 4RN

Routledge is an imprint of the Taylor & Francis Group, an informa business

First issued in paperback 2012

Cover design by Kathryn Houghtaling Lacey, based on original art by Nicholas Wade

Library of Congress Cataloging-in-Publication Data

Wade, Nicholas.
Purkinje's vision : the dawning of neuroscience / by Nicholas J. Wade and Josef Brožek, in collaboration with Jiří Hoskovec.
p. cm.
Includes bibliographical references and index.
ISBN 0-8058-3642-X (cloth : alk. paper)
1. Purkyně, Jan Evangelista, 1787–1869 2. Neuroscientists—Biography. 3. Vision—Research—History. I. Brožek, Josef. II. Hoskovec, Jiří. III. Title.

QP475 .W244 2001
612.8′092—dc21
[B] 00-065416

10 9 8 7 6 5 4 3 2 1

ISBN: 9780415651219 (pbk)

Dedicated to
Christine and Eunice

Contents

Preface xi

1 Introduction **1**

Vision 3

Accommodation 5

Strabismus 10

Direct and Indirect Vision 11

Purkinje Shift 13

Motion Aftereffects 14

Vertigo 15

Neuroscience 23

Psychology 26

2 Biographical and Bibliographical Notes **29**

Early life 29

Purkinje's Views of Psychology 33

Psychological Contributions During the Breslau Years 33

Objective Psychology 35

Return to Prague 36

Additional Contributions 37

Opera Omnia 37

3 Historical Background for Research in Subjective Visual Phenomena **41**

Introduction 41

Light and Shade Figures (I) 42

Pressure Figures (II, III, and XXII) 44

Galvanic Light Phenomena (IV) 46

Intrinsic Light and Ganzfeld Effects (V and VII) 47

Interocular Light Effects (VI) 47

Blind Spot (VIII, X, and XI) 48
Pattern Disappearances With Steady Fixation Outside the Blind Spot (IX) 49
Light Halos (XII) 50
Retinal Blood Vessels (The Purkinje Tree) (XIII) 50
Afterimages and Visual Persistence (XIV) 51
Pattern Distortions (XV–XVII) 55
Voluntary Movement of the Pupil (XVIII) 56
Entoptic Phenomena (XIX–XXI and XXIII) 57
Firey Rings (XXIV) 58
Single and Double Vision (XXV) 58
Staring Vaguely into the Distance (XXVI) 59
Eye Movements (XXVII) 60
Imagination and Memory Images (XXVIII) 62

4 Observations and Experiments on the Physiology of the Senses. Contributions to the Knowledge of Vision in Its Subjective Aspect 65

I. Light and Shade Figures 68
II. Pressure Figures 71
III. Appearance of the Previous Figure under Other Conditions. Clarification Experiment 74
IV. Galvanic Light Figures 77
V. Wandering Cloudy Stripes 79
VI. A Light Phenomenon in the Dark Field of My Right Eye During Increased Activity of the Left Eye 81
VII. Scintillating Light Points When Viewing a White Surface. Spontaneous Spots of Light in the Visual Field 82
VIII. The Place of Entry of the Optic Nerve 82
IX. Disappearance of Objects Outside the Entry of the Optic Nerve 84
X. The Entry Point of the Optic Nerve Visible as a Luminous Circle 85
XI. Appearance of Light at the Entry of the Optic Nerve 86
XII. Halos 87
XIII. Vascular Patterns of the Eye 87
XIV. Afterimages 88
XV. Cloudy Streaks While Viewing Parallel Lines 92
XVI. Zigzag Scintillations Following Observation of Parallel Lines 94

XVII. Changes of Parallel Straight Lines into Wavy Lines 94
XVIII. Voluntary Movement of the Pupil 95
XIX. A Spot in the Middle of the Visual Field During Strenuous Near Fixation 95
XX. Visibility of Blood Circulation in the Eye 96
XXI. Flying Gnats 96
XXII. Curvilinear Star Pattern 98
XXIII. A Pulsating Figure 99
XXIV. Luminous Rings 100
XXV. Unity of the Two Visual Fields. Double Vision 102
XXVI. Staring Vaguely into the Distance 104
XXVII. Eye Movements 105
XXVIII. Persisting Images, Imagination, and Visual Memory 107

5 Assessment **111**
Neuroscience 114
Vertigo 116
Vision 118

References **129**
Name Index **141**
Subject Index **145**

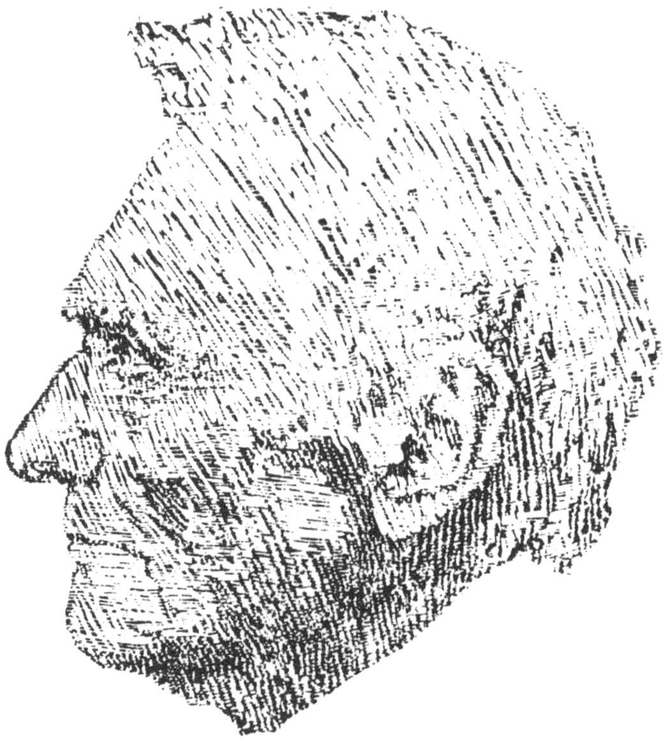

FRONTISPIECE. Jan Evangelista Purkinje (1787–1869) after a frontispiece illustration in Purkinje's *Opera Omnia*, volume 1.

Preface

The life of Jan Evangelista Purkinje (1787–1869) has fascinated students from many disciplines. Histologists marvel at his early descriptions of cells, physiologists admire his attempts to relate structure to function, pharmacologists view in awe his heroic experiments on self-administered drugs, forensic scientists acknowledge his role in the use of fingerprints for identification, and Czech patriots salute his awakening of pride in their nation. Yet all these achievements followed his initial enquiries into vision. It is this psychological dimension that fostered our collaboration, because it is the discipline from which we both come. In his doctoral dissertation Purkinje sought to describe a range subjective visual phenomena and to account for them in objective terms. His dissertation was published in German in 1819 and reprinted in 1823. Surprisingly, it has not been translated into English, and it was this situation we wished to remedy.

As the title suggests, the present volume is bifocal. In the narrow sense it refers to Purkinje's studies of vision, but in its broader view it concerns Purkinje's anticipation of neuroscience. We think of neuroscience as a modern discipline, but its origins are ancient. Purkinje provided evidence to support both its cellular and its conceptual base. At the cellular level his acute vision is immortalized within our bodies, with Purkinje cells in the celebellum and Purkinje fibers surrounding the heart. At the conceptual level, he sought to relate subjective phenomena to their objective underpinnings—to link psychology to physiology. Toward the end of his life he mused on this relationship: "As yet, a rigorously empirical psychology does not exist. It can be developed only *more physiologico*, by comparing systematically the vital phenomena accessible to introspection with the organismic phenomena . . . . Much may be expected from the newer neurology, combined with rigorously empirical introspective observations. The phenomena accessible to the inner sense can be ascertained with the same dependability as the phenomena studied by using the external senses" (Brožek & Hoskovec, 1987, p. 118).

Vision provides a bond that unites psychology and physiology, and it is this bond that was strengthened by Purkinje's enquiries. He was an observer par excellence, and several visual phenomena bear his name—the Purkinje shift, Purkinje images, and the Purkinje tree. However, the breadth of his vision did not always permit scrutiny of the history of the phenomena he described. We have tried to provide a context in which Purkinje's descriptions of visual phenomena can be placed. In some cases this exposes clear precursors of research for which Purkinje has been credited originality, as in the case of his experiments on visual vertigo. In others, there was nothing to suggest the phenomena that he exposed.

Our backgrounds are in psychology, but the path to our collaboration was an unexpected one. Some years ago, one of us published a book, entitled *Psychologists in Word and Image*, which the other was asked to review for a journal. Purkinje was, of course, one of those psychologists who were accorded a "perceptual portrait." In the course of subsequent correspondence it transpired that we had both commenced translating Purkinje's first book on subjective vision, but neither of us had pursued it to its conclusion. Our reasons differed: In one case it was due to a lack of confidence in translating somewhat archaic German; in the other it was because of doubts about knowledge of the history of vision. Accordingly, the prospect of conflating our ignorances was attractive, and we proceeded with the project. It might well have disappeared into one of Purkinje's "wandering cloudy stripes" had it not been for Emily Wilkinson and her colleagues at Lawrence Erlbaum Associates, who offered both encouragement and a contract!

Purkinje was born in Bohemia and his native language was Czech. He used this German version of his name in most of his scientific publications, reverting to the Czech Purkyně after his return to Prague. He is referred to increasingly as Purkyně in modern treatments of his work. However, the book translated here was published under the name Purkinje, and so we have used the Germanic version throughout the text.

Writing a book about a giant of Czech science without contact with the seat to which Purkinje returned (Charles University, Prague) would have been difficult. We have been richly rewarded in this regard by collaboration with Professor Jiří Hoskovec, who has provided essential biographical and pictorial material pertaining to Purkinje. The book has many more illustrations than was initially envisaged, thanks to Professor Hoskovec. Each chapter starts and ends with an illustration relevant to the material covered; these are mostly, but not always, portraits.

Collaborating over continents can present problems, but these were greatly reduced by Margaret Caliandro, who most kindly transcribed the translated text of chapter 4 into computer format.

Producing the book has been encouraged and endured by our wives, to whom it is dedicated.

Nicholas J. Wade
Newport-on-Tay
December 2000

Josef Brožek
Saint Paul

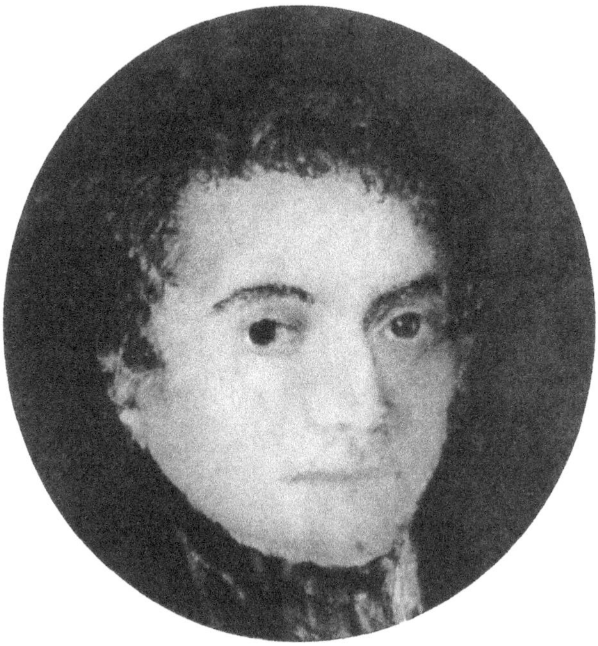

FIG. 1.1. Portrait of Purkinje as a young man (after an illustration in Psotníčková, 1955).

1

Introduction

It is an imperative belief of the natural scientist that each and every modification of a subjective state in the sphere of the senses corresponds to an objective state.

—Purkinje (1819, 1823a, p. 92)

Dawn heralds a transformation of vision. The brightnesses of colors change differentially: Blue objects that appeared brighter than red ones before sunrise reverse thereafter. This phenomenon must have been seen throughout the history of humankind, but Purkinje observed it and committed it to print in 1825. It is now called the Purkinje shift, and it can be related to the different spectral sensitivities of rod and cone receptors in the retina. Purkinje created a shift in more than our appreciation of colors: He shifted the way in which we think about vision itself and of the links with our underlying biology. His vision was that all subjective experiences have objective correlates. This was the dawn of neuroscience.

In the quest to achieve his vision, Jan Evangelista Purkinje or Purkyně (1787–1869) left his mark throughout the body. There are Purkinje cells in the brain, Purkinje fibers around the heart, Purkinje images are reflected from the optical surfaces of the eye, a Purkinje tree (the shadows of the retinal blood vessels) can be rendered visible, and at dawn and dusk we can experience the Purkinje shift. As a medical student, he investigated subjective visual phenomena in part because he did not have access to any physiological apparatus, but also because he believed that visual illusions revealed visual truths.

Purkinje's interests in vision were stimulated by reading Goethe's (1810) *Zur Farbenlehre* (*Theory of Colors*) as a medical student (Grüsser, 1984; Kruta, 1966). Goethe's theory was founded on phenomenological descriptions of perceptual experience, and he rejected the physicalism of Newton's (1704) and Young's (1802) theories. Goethe championed the alternative approach based on color experience rather than color mixing. Newton stated that "the Rays to speak properly are not coloured" (1704, p. 90), thus accepting the subjective dimension in color vision, but he did not subordinate the physics of light to the philosophy of sight in the manner of Goethe. One of Goethe's greatest difficulties was reconciling the purity of the perception of white light with the conception of its compound nature. However, he was able to enlist a variety of phenomena (such as color contrasts, color shadows, accidental colors, and aspects of color blindness) that posed severe difficulties for the trichromatic theory of Young (1802) and later of Helmholtz (1867, 2000b). Despite the wealth of observations contained in his *Theory of Colors*, few students of vision saw Goethe's theory as other than evidence of the distance that separated art from science. In a lecture surveying Goethe's scientific researches, Helmholtz attempted to take a sympathetic view by stating that he was primarily a poet and that he was not disposed to support experimental enquiries into natural phenomena: "Thus, in the theory of colour, Goethe remains faithful to his principle, that Nature must reveal her secrets of her own free will; that she is but the transparent representation of the ideal world" (Helmholtz, 1898, p. 45).

Goethe sought to shift the study of color vision away from physics toward phenomenology. Accordingly, he was impressed by the publication, in 1819, of Purkinje's *Beiträge zur Kenntniss des Sehens in subjectiver Hinsicht* (*Contributions to the Knowledge of Vision in its Subjective Aspect*) and saw him as an advocate of the phenomenological method, although Goethe did display disappointment that his own observations were not cited by Purkinje (see Kruta, 1966). Later Goethe encouraged Purkinje's academic career, although he did not receive the unstinting support from Purkinje that he probably expected. Purkinje acknowledged Goethe's influence but retained an independent theoretical standpoint. Whereas Goethe had attempted to replace physicalism with phenomenology, Purkinje sought to emphasize the physiological dimension of perception.

Purkinje's second book on subjective visual phenomena (1825a) was dedicated to Goethe. When Purkinje gained access to one of the new large achromatic microscopes, in the early 1830s, he put his observational skills to good use, as is attested by the Purkinje cells in the brain and the Purkinje fibers in the heart. The laboratory in Breslau where he conducted these microscopical studies has been referred to as "the cradle of histology," and his research was a significant contribution to the development of cell theory and the neuron doctrine. Thus Purkinje provided not only the conceptual foundations for neuroscience but also the building blocks for its construction. His vision did herald the dawning of neuroscience.

VISION

The 19th century witnessed a revolution in the study of vision—it was displaced from the natural environment and transferred to the laboratory. The study of vision was transformed from an observational to an experimental discipline after 1840 (see Wade, 1998a). The seeds of the revolution were sown much earlier—in the 17th century—with an appreciation of the physical nature of light and of the anatomical structure of the eye. Kepler (1604, 1611) described the manner in which light is refracted through the eye to form an image on the retina, and Scheiner (1619) provided an accurate representation of the anatomy of the eye. Both Kepler and Scheiner constructed artificial eyes so that the nature of image formation could be examined more systematically (see Park, 1997; Wade, 1998c). The analogy between eye and camera focused interest on the geometrical properties of the retinal image and on the ways in which two retinal images could be combined. This concern with spatial vision was replaced with the investigation of color phenomena in the 18th century, largely as a consequence of Newton's (1704) analysis of the visible spectrum. Isolating and mixing light of different colors did lend some degree of experimental control to the study of vision, but it generally remained an observational rather than an experimental pursuit.

In the 18th century, physics had made advances by isolating variables and then manipulating them, and much the same applied to the study of vision in the 19th century. Questions about the nature of vision have been asked since antiquity. For example, why do we perceive the world the way that we do, and how does this come about? In this context the nature of space and time was a central issue in philosophical discussions. Toward the end of the 18th century, Kant (1781) declared space and time to be a priori dimensions and thus objects of transcendental aesthetics. This represented a fundamental distinction between his position and that of contemporary empiricist philosophers, like Hume. From Kant's standpoint the perception of space and time was outside the realm of experimental enquiry. The natural scientists of the early 19th century demonstrated, on the other hand, that instruments could be devised that enabled the manipulation of perceived space and time (see Wade & Heller, 1997). The most important of these instruments were the stroboscope, the stereoscope, and the chronoscope; the stroboscope varied space and time together, whereas the other two instruments provided a means for the analysis of space and time separately. Moreover, these instruments proved, contrary to Kant's (1786) assertion, that the study of vision could indeed be scientific. There existed a body of observations concerning phenomena that could be experienced in the natural environment, but there was little in the way of controlling or manipulating the conditions under which they could be seen. This was made possible by the use of the various scopes, and the methods of physics could be applied to the measurements of the senses.

Despite the grand design behind Purkinje's vision, his initial experimental work was based on observations of visual phenomena that were made without any elaborate equipment. His studies of vision were conducted before the instrumental revolution took place, and he extended the range of phenomena that can be experienced in the natural environment. The slim volume *Beiträge zur Kenntniss des Sehens in subjectiver Hinsicht* was his doctoral dissertation, which was defended in 1818 and published in 1819. It was reprinted in 1823 with a prefix to the title: *Beobachtungen und Versuche zur Physiologie der Sinne* (*Observations and Experiments on the Physiology of the Senses*) (1823a). The book had a major impact on sensory physiology in Germany, and the phenomena it described continue to be investigated today. Purkinje defined and named a new area of study—subjective visual phenomena. This was taken by Goethe to emphasize the subjective dimension of all vision, but Purkinje himself sought to determine the objective correlates of the subjective impressions. In so doing, he set in train the tradition that finds expression in contemporary neuroscience—relating aspects of our experience to their underlying physiological foundations.

Purkinje's book, which is translated in chapter 4, described a range of subjective impressions, some of which were novel and others of which were steeped in antiquity. Purkinje himself was parsimonious in the references he cited, perhaps because at that early stage of his career he was unaware of the wider literature. Grüsser (1984) suggested that Purkinje had access to books on vision by Darwin (1795), Goethe (1810), and Steinbuch (1811). Thus Purkinje was unlikely to have been inhibited in his observations by a burden of received wisdom; this is one of the reasons for the freshness of his descriptions of visual phenomena.

Erasmus Darwin's *Zoonomia* was translated into German soon after its publication in English. It provided a survey of the senses from a physiological point of view and related all functions in health and sickness to irritability, sensitivity, volition, and association, and these in turn were discussed in terms of motions of the body parts. Darwin argued by analogy and made many shrewd observations of perception. He commenced his treatise with a statement of intent: "The purport of the following pages is an endeavour to reduce the facts belonging to animal life into classes, orders, genera, and species; and by comparing them with each other, to unravel the theory of diseases" (1794, p. 1). Purkinje was particularly influenced by Darwin's speculations on vertigo.

Goethe's *Theory of Colors* (1810) presented an attack on the physicalism of Newtonian optics by emphasizing the purity of white light and stressing the subjective dimension of color perception. In line with many Romantic philosophers, Goethe rejected the experimental approach to the study of nature because it was too constrained. In its place he proposed the astute and intuitive observation of natural phenomena, setting in train the method of phenomenology. In the context of color vision, he based his theory on color experience rather than color mixing, and he championed the philosophy of sight rather than the physics of light. Steinbuch's *Beytrag zur Physiologie der Sinne* (*Contribution to the Physiology of the Senses*) (1811) was also influenced by Darwin's *Zoonomia* and tried to integrate the psychology of perception with its underlying physiology (see Hatfield,

1990). Steinbuch developed an empiricist and associationist theory of spatial perception based on muscular activity, and he expressed a sentiment linking subjective experience to objective stimulation that is echoed in Purkinje's work.

There was much research on some subjective visual phenomena before that of Purkinje, and this is sketched in chapter 3. The aim of the present section is to describe some of the additional aspects of vision that he examined in his early years. It is clear that vision was not only his initial but also his abiding scientific interest. Much of the work following his doctoral dissertation was on vision, most particularly a long article on vertigo (Purkinje, 1820) and coverage of a range of visual phenomena in his inaugural lecture at the University of Breslau (Purkinje, 1823b). The inaugural lecture referred to his research on accommodation, peripheral vision, and long and short sightedness, and he addressed all these issues in his book of *Neue Beiträge* (*New Contributions*) (Purkinje, 1825a). It is these topics that are dealt with initially, together with strabismus, the Purkinje shift, and motion aftereffects; a separate section is devoted to his experiments on vertigo.

Accommodation

The manner in which the eye could focus on objects at different distances was a source of much debate and one to which the Purkinje images reflected from the surfaces of the cornea and lens was to assist in solving. This is called the problem of accommodation, the term that was coined by Porterfield (1738). From the time of Kepler to the middle of the 19th century, accommodation was one of the most intensively studied and controversial topics in vision. Before Purkinje's work, Priestley (1772) noted: "That we are capable of viewing objects with nearly equal distinctness, though they are placed at considerably different distances, is evident; but the alteration that takes place in the eye for this purpose, or the mechanism by which this effect is produced, is not easily ascertained" (p. 638). Helmholtz, who was to provide the solution, summarized the situation thus: "The mechanism by which this is accomplished . . . was one of the greatest riddles of the physiology of the eye since the time of Kepler . . . . No problem in optics has given rise to so many contradictory theories as this" (1873, p. 205).

At the beginning of the 19th century the major candidate mechanisms for accommodation had long been known. Kepler (1611) proposed that the lens moved forward and backward in the eye itself; Scheiner (1619) observed pupil contraction when the eye focused on near objects; Descartes (1637) speculated that the lens changed in curvature; Rohault (1671) entertained the possibility that the eye could lengthen or shorten; and Desaguliers (1719) suggested that the corneal curvature was increased when the eye viewed near objects. In addition to these theories, La Hire (1685a, 1685b) argued that there is no active process of accommodation because of pupil constriction when the eye is viewing near objects and the ability to ignore blurred images. Although Scheiner observed the constriction of the pupil with fixation on near objects, he still inclined toward Kepler's view that the lens moved in the eye. He did, however, entertain the possibility that the lens could become more convex.

William Porterfield (1738) and William Charles Wells (1792) carried out the most systematic experiments on accommodation before those of Thomas Young (1793, 1801) and Purkinje (see Wade, 2000a). Porterfield devised and named an instrument called an optometer for determining the near and the far points of vision, and he was able to discount hypotheses based on the fixed curvature of the crystalline lens by recourse to sight following its removal. He examined such an aphakic individual who was unable to accommodate at all without the aid of a convex lens, the power of which was required to be modified for objects at different distances (see Wade, 1998a, 1998c). Porterfield concluded that, because elongation of the eye was still possible for such a person, as was variation in corneal curvature, the crystalline lens must be involved in accommodation. Nonetheless, Porterfield remained unsure of the mechanism of lenticular function. The involvement of the ciliary process was acknowledged, but its location led him to the conclusion that its action moved the lens forward and backward in the eye. Moreover, it was believed that any changes in the shape of the lens would be a consequence of muscular action within it, the evidence for which was wanting.

Porterfield's optometer consisted of a metal plate with two narrow and close vertical slits in it so that when it was held close to the eye their separation was less than the pupil diameter. The stimulus viewed was a vertical slit illuminated by a candle in a lamp housing; he also tried a black line on white card and a white line on a black card, but these were not so appropriate for distant viewing. The distance of the vertical light line from the vertical slits could be changed so that the near and the far points of vision could be measured, that is, the nearest and the farthest positions at which the line could be seen as single; variations in pupil diameter were not controlled. Young (1801) improved on Porterfield's optometer by incorporating a lens and a graduated scale.

Wells (1792) developed an alternative method for determining the near and the far points of vision—the image of a candle flame reflected from the bulb of a small thermometer. With this he determined the different ranges of distinct vision for his own left and right eyes and the intermediate accommodation that attends binocular viewing of objects within the range of one eye but not the other. Purkinje (1823b) referred to yet another technique (in standard use by opticians at the time) involving a graduated scale along which letters could be presented.

Despite the force of all the arguments for the involvement of the lens in accommodation, its mechanism of action remained a mystery. Following Young's (1793) proposal that the curvature of the lens changes, Wells (1811) remarked that he had attempted to observe such variations in 1794 "by applying to the crystallines of oxen, which had been felled from thirty seconds to a minute before, chemical and mechanical stimuli, and those of Galvanism and electricity; but in no instance was any alteration of figure, or other indication of muscular power, observed" (p. 390). It was still anticipated that change in the shape of the lens could be effected only by muscular activity within the lens itself, and no evidence of muscular components could be found. Accordingly, the accepted conclusion was that the lens moved forward or backward within the eye.

Both Wells (1811) and Purkinje (1825a) examined the effects of belladonna on vision, and in this case a translation of Wells' article into German (Wells, 1813) was cited by Purkinje. Wells had conducted experiments on his own vision two decades earlier but he was unable to make further experiments because by 1811 his eyesight had deteriorated markedly. He enlisted the help of a colleague:

> Having discovered that my own eyes were unfit for the experiments, which I wished to make with Belladonna, I instructed an ingenious young physician, Dr. Cutting, from the Island of Barbadoes, and now residing there, in the manner elsewhere described by me, of ascertaining the range of perfect vision by means of luminous points. This he found, in consequence, to begin, with respect to his left eye, at the distance of six inches, and not to terminate at the distance of eight feet, beyond which he could not see clearly the object, with which he had hitherto made his experiments, the image of the flame of a candle in the bulb of a small thermometer. The flame of a lamp, distant about sixty yards, gave a faint indication of its rays meeting before they fell on the retina; the rays from a star had very evidently their focus a little before the membrane. He now applied the juice of Belladonna to his left eye. Half an hour later, when his pupil was but little dilated, perfect vision commenced at the distance of seven inches; in fifteen minutes more, it began at the distance of three feet and a half. When his pupil had acquired its greatest enlargement, the rays from the image of the flame of a candle, in the bulb of a small thermometer at a distance of eight feet, could not be prevented from converging to a point behind the retina. The rays from lamps still more distant, and from stars, had their focuses at the same time on the retina. This state of vision continued, in its greatest extent, to the following day; and it was not till the ninth day after the application of Belladonna, that he completely recovered the power of adapting his eye to near objects. While his left eye was thus affected, the vision of his right eye remained unaltered. (1811, pp. 382–383)

Cutting remarked that the gradual recovery of pupil contraction was not in synchrony with that of accommodation. He repeated the experiment on his right eye, with the same outcome. Even though the effects of certain plant extracts on pupil dilation had been known to the ancients, their effects on accommodation were first described by Wells "with wonderful accuracy" (Donders, 1864, p. 591). Pliny the Elder, in the first century, described how an ointment made from plant extract and honey could be used to dilate the pupil before an operation for cataract (see Pliny 77/1940).

Purkinje (1825a) addressed at length the effects of belladonna on vision in the final section of his *New Contributions*. He initially measured the near and the far points of vision in his right eye, before and 2 hours after the application of belladonna, by using printed letters. He repeated the experiment with Wells' thermometer method for determining the near and the far points and obtained similar results—the near point receded and the range of distinct vision compressed—and they were not affected by converging or diverging the eyes. He attributed the effects to the absence of variation in the curvature of the lens. Purkinje also observed the effects of belladonna on chromatic aberration and on the extent of peripheral vision.

Purkinje's (1823b) earlier demonstration of reflections from the optical surfaces of the eye provided evidence of changes in the curvature of the lens. He wrote:

> If we place the candlelight about six inches from someone's eye in order that we can see the flame on the cornea when we are sitting to the side of the visual axis of the eye, within the circle of the pupil nearer the periphery, we will see in the back of the pupil a blinking flame, still smaller in its diameter but reversed and of feeble illumination, which we can easily judge, by comparing it with the one on the artificial lens, that it is reflected from the posterior wall of the lens. The front surface of the lens, and partly its inner matter, under the conditions of full transparency we can make accessible for observation if, by looking into the pupil from the side and by placing the light on the opposite side of the eye, the straight lines from the eye to the observer and from the light of the candle shining into the pupil form an obtuse angle. Here one will see an elongated image of the flame, which, because it is straight, shows that it is reflected from the convex surface of the lens . . . . Both of these methods for the observation of the surfaces of the lens will not be without use, I think, in therapeutic investigation, especially where one wants to differentiate precisely whether only the capsule of the lens is involved, the lens itself, its posterior surface, or the vitreous humor. From the exact measurements of the flame reflections on the lens of a living human subject one can determine with considerable labor its shape and its relation to the acuity of vision. (John, 1959, p. 59)

The drawings of the reflections are shown in Fig. 1.2.

Accommodation, of course, is linked to the difficulties that some individuals have in focusing on near and far objects, that is, the errors of refraction that are widespread in the population. Interest in the history of eye corrections for such errors derives from the use of optical instruments as aids to scientific enquiry (Crombie, 1967; Singer, 1921). Telescopes and microscopes use the same basic materials, ground-glass lenses, to explore the upper and the lower limits of nature inaccessible to the naked eye. Yet there was a long period before the connection between eyeglasses and other optical instruments was made. Historical accounts of the development of eyeglasses themselves can be found in Hill (1915), Needham and Gwei-Djen (1967), Rosen (1956a, 1956b), and Schmitz (1982, 1995).

The fact that individuals differed in the visual detail that they could discriminate was remarked on by Aristotle (Ross, 1927) and Pliny (77/1940). Moreover, Seneca (63/1971) gave an account of the magnification of letters seen through a lens or a burning glass (a water-filled glass ball). Weakness of vision in short-sighted and older people was commented on by Aristotle, who speculated that they might have different foundations: the former inspected objects at close distances whereas the latter viewed them from afar. He also noted that short-sighted people reduced the aperture of the pupil in order to see more clearly. In addition to these individual

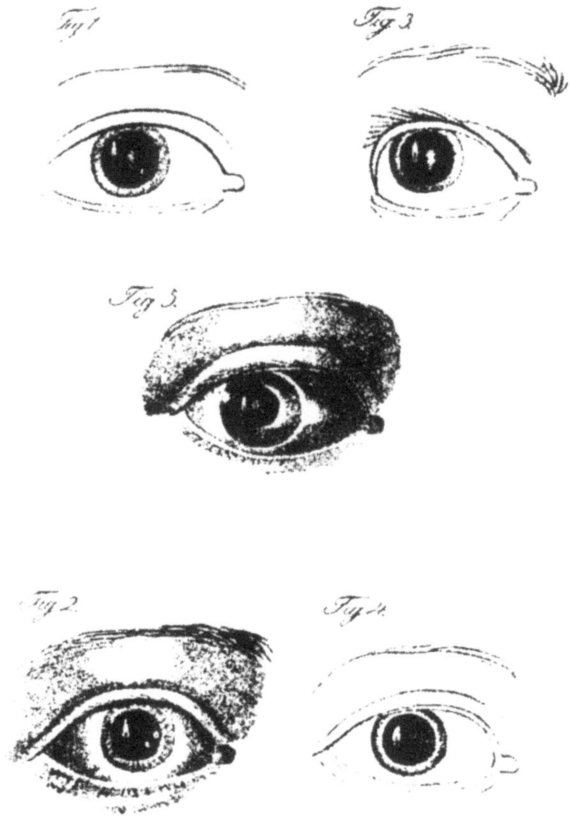

FIG. 1.2. Purkinje images. The reflections of a candle flame from the structures of the eye, from Purkinje (1823b): "Fig. 1. Candlelight reflection from anterior and posterior cornea and from the anterior and posterior portion of the lens. Fig. 2. Candlelight reflection from the anterior surface of the cornea and the posterior surface of the lens where the image is reversed. Fig. 3. Candlelight reflection from the anterior surface of the cornea and from the anterior surface of the lens where the reflection is erect. Fig. 4. Semicircular umbrula (weak shadow) which projects from the iris to the anterior surface of the lens. Fig. 5. A light from the substantia albuginea to the center of the anterior chamber" (John, 1959, p. 61).

differences, Purkinje was acutely aware of differences between the eyes within an individual. He commented on the weakness of his left eye with respect to his right, and many of his observations were restricted to his better right eye.

Optical corrections for presbyopia are considered to have been adopted from the late 13th century, initially by Roger Bacon, and thereafter avidly exploited by many, and there was an element of the magical or the mercenary in their production. The inscription on a burial slab in Florence, marking the death of one Salvino degli Armati in 1317, noted that he was the inventor of eyeglasses, for which God was asked to forgive him his sins! Eyeglasses were soon depicted in paintings, the earliest of which is said to be by Tommaso da Modena in 1352 (Rosen, 1956a; Schmitz, 1982, 1995). Maurolico (1611) came much closer to appreciating the correct relationship; while still maintaining that the crystalline lens was the receptive organ, he described changes in its shape and associated these changes with myopia and presbyopia. Moreover, he advocated the use of concave lenses for short-sighted eyes, in contrast to convex lenses for older eyes.

Thus, although the assistance of convex lenses in presbyopia was readily appreciated in the 13th century, the integration of the lenticular optics with vision and their relation to accommodation was to wait another three centuries. Two factors retarded such integration: ignorance of both the dioptrics and the anatomy of the eye. When these were more clearly understood, early in the 17th century, corrections for both short and long sightedness became routine, notwithstanding the doubts that remained concerning their causes. Kepler (1604) considered that these conditions were a consequence of experience; those whose work involved detailed observation of near objects became incapable of seeing distant objects, and vice versa. Descartes (1637/1902) analysis was much more mechanistic and pragmatic. He attributed short and long sightedness to the shape of the eyeball itself and sought to determine the appropriate optical correction by essentially using different lenses to define the near and the far points of distinct vision.

Thereafter the corrections for myopia and presbyopia were amplified and illustrated by many writers (see Wade, 1998a). Bifocal glasses were introduced by Benjamin Franklin (1785): Because reading was normally accomplished with a downward gaze and scanning the scenery with an upward gaze, the two halves of the spectacles could be so constructed to accommodate both functions.

Strabismus

Distortion of the eyes (strabismus) was recorded in the Ebers papyrus over 3,000 years ago, but its reported association with problems of binocular vision are more recent (see Hirschberg, 1899; Shastid, 1917; Duke-Elder & Wybar, 1973). Aristotle (Ross, 1927) described the ensuing double vision, and Galen (May, 1968) noted that the deviations of the eyes were always nasal or temporal; however, Galen also stated that strabismics rarely make errors in object recognition. Corrections for the deviation were advocated by Paul of Ægineta (680/1844): He recommended the use of a mask that has also been attributed to Paré (1564). The most elaborate masks were prescribed by Bartisch (1583), who appreciated that strabismus was more amenable to correction in children than in adults. Jurin (1738) and Reid (1764) sought to strengthen the weaker eye by exercise, and Bell (1803) suggested patching the stronger eye.

From the 18th century, attention was directed to the manner in which strabismics saw objects singly. There were those like Jurin, Reid, and Bell who believed that the nondeviating eye suppressed the signals from the deviating one. This was so despite the opposite's being maintained by the strabismics themselves. The suppression could be a consequence of muscular misalignment or a refractive difference between the eyes. Others, like Hartley (1749) and Harris (1775), considered that the new pattern of stimulation could be learned (by association) to yield singleness of vision. Hartley stated that the origin of the deviation lay in the asymmetrical cradling of children. Reid raised 11 theoretical queries about strabismus and also had some success at training strabismics to bifixate on objects.

Studies of strabismus epitomize the emphasis that has been placed on binocular single vision; the many comparisons that were made between strabismic and binocular individuals dwelt on this to the exclusion of other aspects of binocular vision, like stereopsis. Purkinje (1825a) was perhaps reflecting on his own eyesight when he stated that "It is true that in almost all squinters one eye is weaker than the other, or more often one is shortsighted and the other longsighted . . . the shortsighted eye alone and exclusively turns inwards in order, so to speak, to disregard the object" (p. 165). He also speculated that a weak and amblyopic eye will tend to be passive and unmoving (relative to movements of the stronger eye) so that the strabismus might not appear so marked. However, he did distinguish among convergent, parallel, and divergent forms of strabismus, and he described the effects of "voluntary squinting" or viewing objects with asymmetrical vergence.

Direct and Indirect Vision

The term distinct vision had long been used to describe the superior visual acuity in the visual axis. Indeed, Euclid (ca. 300 B.C.; see Burton, 1945) related distinct vision to visual acuity and gave an instance of sharply defined corners appearing rounded when viewed from a distance. In like manner, Ptolemy (ca. 150; see Smith, 1996) provided a general statement regarding the greater distinctiveness of vision along the axis of the eye as opposed to more lateral rays. He accounted for this by saying that perpendicular rays were stronger than oblique ones, and an empirical demonstration of distinct vision was given by Ibn al-Haytham or Alhazen (ca. 1040; see Sabra, 1989). He used a board extended in front of the observer's eyes and fixed two equivalently written words in central and peripheral locations; the central word was more easily read than the lateral one. The indistinctness of the lateral word increased with movement into the periphery. The experiment was conducted with monocular and binocular observation with essentially the same results. Few measured the range of direct vision, but Harris (1775) gave an astute estimate of the size of the field of distinct vision, namely, a visual angle of 1°–2°. Harris also estimated the extent of the visual field, providing values of 60° in all directions from the point of fixation.

The first topic addressed by Purkinje (1825a) in his *New Contributions* was indirect or peripheral vision. Ptolemy and Ibn al-Haytham discussed distinct and peripheral vision together, and the latter conducted experiments by using written words as stimuli extending into peripheral vision; he determined how far letters needed to be moved peripherally before they became illegible (see Sabra, 1989). The magnitudes of these extents were not given, and many centuries were to pass before values were derived. Purkinje did make reference to Young's (1801) estimates of the limits of the visual fields, although he neglected to mention those of Harris (1775). Purkinje was able to make more precise estimates because he devised a simple perimeter with which to make measurements. The rudiments of this instrument were described in his inaugural lecture at Breslau in 1823:

> In the visual field there is a point in the line of vision where the vision is more distinct than elsewhere. If the visual line terminates in this point we call it direct vision. Indirect vision is the viewing of all other points in the visual field which are outside the visual axis and are seen indistinctly and obliquely.... To observe the extent of direct vision more precisely, compose a segment of three-quarters of a circle divided into degrees, from the center of which the eye, without the movement of the head, can look at a picture which is distinctly seen when moved on the circle's circumference. Let the observer report how far he sees it clearly, that is, until the limitation of the eyeball's movement is reached, when it will be necessary to stop the picture on the periphery and to note the angle in degrees through which the eye moved when the picture was moved to the side.... The extension of indirect vision is given by the space which is less clearly seen when the eye is fixed on one point in the visual field. To determine the range of the extension of indirect vision the apparatus of the preceding experiment can be used, a target being added on which the eye is fixed, while a second, well-illuminated target is moved in or out from the side. (John, 1959, pp. 57–58)

Purkinje used the perimeter not only to determine the dimensions of the visual field but also to define the limits of color discrimination in the eye: "My measurements of the width of indirect vision indicate a temporal angle of 100 degrees (extended to 115 degrees when the pupil is enlarged by belladonna), 80 degrees downwards, 60 degrees upwards, and the same value for the nasal angle" (1825a, p. 6). Purkinje emphasized the importance of peripheral vision generally, and more specifically with regard to detecting movement of objects, by means of a simple viewing tube with a small aperture so that peripheral vision was excluded.

It was not until Purkinje's specification of color zones that serious attention was directed to variations of color perception within individuals. With the perimeter, colored squares could be moved systematically toward the point of fixation. At the edges of the visual field, over 90° from the fixation point, objects were barely visible and rapidly disappeared from view. Moving to more central locations, the object first became visible and only later appeared colored. He found that yellow and blue were visible at slightly greater peripheral angles than red and green and that all colors were visible more peripherally in the temporal than in the nasal fields. His description was as follows (1825a):

> If one moves a colored square slowly at the edge of the graduated curve [a perimeter] from the temporal side towards the point of direct vision, so one has initially only an impression of the shape and color of an undefined something that is moving forwards. Every effort to distinguish the shape makes the object disappear completely; it disappears just as quickly when one fixes the attention on the point of direct vision. This occurs at an angle (to the temporal side) of 110–90 degrees. Below 90 degrees the color quality and the shape begin to become noticeable, but still very uncertainly. However, in the case of the color it appears more generally light or dark, as happens in the gradually approaching darkness of evening when the color of the object becomes uncertain. Cinnabar is visible at an angle of 90–70 degrees (temporally) as a very pale yellow, then orange, and then transforms gradually to its true color quality; this is found at a visual angle from 60 degrees inwards; a beautiful pure purple appears black at an outer angle of 90 degree, blue at 80 degrees, violet at 70 degrees, and first begins to take on its true color at 50; light blue looks white at 90 degrees, but assumes its own color at 80 degrees and less; a saturated blue appears as such at its first presentation in the visual field; violet appears black at 90 degrees, blue at 80 and 70 degrees, and first at 60 degrees and less as such in different shades; a saturated green looks black between 90 and 80 degrees after which it starts to develop its own color; light yellow appears as such on its outermost presentation, as does orange; rosy red was initially white, its color emerged first at 70 degrees; a leaf of Origanum majus appears initially dull until 40 degrees, then increasingly brighter yellow, and from there through yellow–green to its own colour. In a nasal direction and also upwards and downwards these color changes take place even earlier, as the visual field itself is more restricted. (pp. 15–16)

Purkinje Shift

Perhaps the most cited observation made in *New Contributions* of 1825 was what we now call the Purkinje shift that can be witnessed at dawn or dusk (1825a):

> The degree of objective illumination has a great influence on the intensity of color quality. In order to prove this most vividly, take some colors before daybreak, when it begins slowly to get lighter. Initially one sees only black and grey. Then the brightest colors, red and green, appear darkest. Yellow cannot be distinguished from a rosy red. Blue looks to me the most noticeable. Nuances of red, which otherwise burn brightest in daylight, namely carmine, cinnabar and orange show themselves as darkest, in contrast to their average brightness. Green appears more bluish, and its yellow tint develops with the increasing daylight. (pp. 109–110)

Another translation of this passage can be found in Brožek (1989); the term "Purkinje phenomenon" was coined by de Lepinay and Nicati in 1882 (see Brožek & Kuthan, 1990; Brožek, Kuthan, and Arens, 1991), and it is also referred to as the Purkinje shift.

Purkinje himself did not attribute great importance to the phenomenon as it was the ninth entry in the section on color combination. Earlier reports of a similar phenomenon can be found in Aristotle and Leonardo da Vinci, although they are by no means as explicit as the clear phenomenological description given by Purkinje (see Wade, 1998a). A shadowy figure in the history of this phenomenon is Mathias Klotz, a Bavarian artist who wrote two books on color theory (Klotz, 1806, 1816). Brožek et al. (1991) discovered, to their surprise, a reference in the 17th edition of *Brockhaus Enzyklopädie* to a description of the phenomenon by Klotz (1816); the author of the entry was anonymous (see Anon, 1972). Klotz commenced *Gründliche Farbenlehre* (*A Comprehensive Theory of Colors*) by regretting the fact that it followed so closely on Goethe's tome and hence was less likely to make an impact. This prediction was indeed accurate as the book has rarely been cited, despite insightful passages on brightness contrast in addition to color changes under varying illumination. As was the case with Purkinje, the color change was noticed by chance; Klotz had been painting a military portrait and noted that some features of the uniform appeared to change color toward dusk. This led him to conduct more controlled observations with patches of colored paper on a neutral background: Red appeared brighter than blue by daylight, with the reverse by twilight: "If one places two discs (each of about three inches diameter), one of blue and the other of red, in the middle of a sheet of grey paper, and compare them by daylight, then the red will appear much brighter than the blue. Thereafter, with approaching twilight, one observes the same discs every two minutes and one will note that the blue loses its colour earlier than the red; then—what is still more remarkable is that the blue appears to lose its darkness—whereas the red gets darker" (Klotz, 1816, p. 19). Unlike Purkinje, Klotz did not base his conclusions on his own observations alone as they were confirmed by a friend!

Motion Aftereffects

In 1820 Purkinje wrote an extensive article on his observations of vertigo (see the next section). In the course of his descriptions of visual motion induced by body rotation he mentioned a type of apparent motion that was dependent on visual stimulation alone. It is now called the motion aftereffect: "Another form of eye dizziness can be demonstrated if one observes a passing sequence of spatially distinct objects for a long time, e.g. a long parade of cavalry, overlapping waves, the spokes of a wheel that is not rotating too fast. When the actual movement of the objects stops there is a similar apparent motion in the opposite direction" (1820, pp. 96–97). He elaborated on this account in the *New Contributions*: "One time I observed a cavalry parade for more than an hour, and then when the parade had passed, the houses directly opposite appeared to me to move in the reversed direction to the parade. While the eye did strive to fixate on each individual row of militia during observation, it moved unconsciously in the same direction as the parade; this movement was repeated so often that it became habitual, and continued when the parade had passed. The eye attempted to fixate on the stationary objects in a similar manner to the motion it had become accustomed to fixating, and therefore glided unconsciously over them in the usual direction, so that the objects appeared to slide away in the opposite direction" (1825a, pp. 60–61).

These were the first reports of the phenomenon for almost 1,900 years. It was described by Aristotle and Lucretius but not by anyone else in the intervening period (see Wade, 1994; Wade & Verstraten, 1998). Thomas Willis (1672) might have been referring to this phenomenon when he discussed vertigo: "Vertigo may also be caused by the sight of a mobile object such as running water because the spirits concerned with vision are caught up in this similar movement" (Dewhurst, 1980, p. 114). The stimulus was appropriate but the report is not precise enough to link it with the motion aftereffect. Erasmus Darwin similarly described the vertiginous effects of viewing rotating and translating motions, but did not mention any aftereffects: "Thus some people become dizzy at the sight of a whirling wheel, or by gazing on the fluctuations of a river, if no steady objects are at the same time within the sphere of distinct vision" (1796, p. 233). Both early descriptions by Aristotle and Lucretius were related to observing stationary objects following exposure to moving water, although Aristotle was not explicit about the direction of the aftereffect. Purkinje provided a clear statement of the direction in which the aftereffect motion was seen—opposite to that of the prior motion. He also suggested an interpretation of it that was to have lasting appeal: During adaptation, the eyes move unconsciously in the direction of motion, and they continue this movement when viewing a stationary object; this would result in their motion with respect to the retina as if they were indeed moving in the opposite direction.

The motion aftereffect is now at the heart of visual neuroscience (see Mather, Verstraten, & Anstis, 1998). Indeed, it could be argued that the phenomenon was in the vanguard of modern research on visual motion. It has been variously called the aftereffect of seen movement, the movement aftereffect, successive motion contrast, and the waterfall illusion. Many of the major figures in visual science in the 19th century, like Müller, Helmholtz, and Mach, added to knowledge about motion aftereffects, and it is now seen as a tool for linking the psychology of vision to its underlying neurophysiology.

VERTIGO

The origins of research on the vestibular system have been attributed to Purkinje and Flourens by historians of the senses. For example, Kornhuber (1974) commenced his survey thus: "The history of vestibular research begins early in the nineteenth century. Against a background of the known anatomical structure of the labyrinth in different animals, the work of Purkinje (1820), Flourens (1824) . . . led to the conclusion that the vestibular end-organs have a different function from hearing, and that they regulate body and eye positions and if disturbed, give rise to vertigo" (p. 3). The situation was described even more graphically by Kruta (1964a): "It is not easy to trace the origins of knowledge in a question of science, but one can say with a tolerably high degree of certainty that the modern origins of the physiology of posture and balance in man and animals starts—after some preliminary work—with that of J. E. Purkyně on vertigo between 1820–1827 and that of M. J. P. Flourens on the functions of different sections of the central nervous system (1822–1824) and the semicircular canals of the inner ear (1824–1828)" (p. 5). Griffith (1922), whose historical survey listed 1,700 articles and books on the vestibular system, commenced with Purkinje and Flourens, with little regard to the earlier research. It is the case that Purkinje held Flourens in very high regard (see Kruta, 1964a, 1964b; Thomsen, 1919), and they were certainly at the forefront of research in this area, but many of Purkinje's experiments on vertigo had been performed over two decades earlier by Wells (see Wade, 2000c).

Vertigo is a disturbance of balance usually accompanied by apparent motion of the surroundings and sometimes with nausea, and it has been a source of interest since antiquity. According to the Roman commentator Diogenes Laertius (1925), in the 4th century B.C., Aristotle's pupil Theophrastus wrote a book on vertigo, but it has not survived. Because it is a condition that accompanies many diseases it has been a source of constant medical interest and speculation. Aristotle (ca. 330 B.C.) described the vertiginous effects of alcohol, Lucretius (ca. 56 B.C.) commented on the consequences of body rotation, and Ptolemy (ca. 150 A.D.) indicated that vertigo could be caused by visual stimulation (see Wade, 1998a). There were sporadic accounts thereafter, but a more systematic approach was taken by Willis (1672), who defined vertigo as "an affection in which visible objects appear to rotate" (p. 353). Willis devoted a chapter to describing its pathology and the conditions that can induce it in healthy individuals. A particular stimulus for vertigo is body rotation, and this, too, was discussed by Willis, who interpreted it Galenic terms. Motion of the animal spirit in the head produced the apparent motion during rotation, rather like smoke in a flask lagging behind that of the rotating vessel. Moreover, Willis described the visual motion that continues after body rotation ceases, and this was attributed to the continued motions of the animal spirit in the head.

Vertigo was often referred to in the 18th century as dizziness or giddiness. Whytt (1765) included giddiness among the symptoms for nervous diseases:

> Many people of a delicate, nervous, and vascular system, after stooping and suddenly raising their head, are apt to be seized with a *vertigo*, which is sometimes accompanied by faintness. In this case, the vessels of the brain being too weak, seem to yield more than usual to the weight of the blood, when the head is inclined; and afterwards, when it is suddenly raised, and the blood at once descends towards the heart, those vessels do not contract fast enough, so as to accommodate themselves to the quantity of blood remaining in them: At the same time the brain, on account of its too great sensibility, is more affected than usual, by any sudden change in the motion of the fluids through its vessels. (p. 309)

Vertigo can be induced by a number of factors like alcohol, looking downward from tall structures, rapid head movement, or body rotation. Erasmus Darwin (1801b) listed the diseases with which vertigo was associated. As indicated above, these effects had been reported repeatedly since antiquity, but Purkinje added order and precision to their classification. He published a long article on vertigo in 1820, and it was followed by several other shorter reports. In 1826 he reviewed Flourens' (1824) book on the effects of cerebellar lesions on postural control and in this and a later article (Purkinje, 1827a) sought to confirm and integrate Flourens' findings with his subjective studies of vertigo. The phenomenon was also addressed briefly in Purkinje's *New Contributions* in the section on real and apparent motion. He distinguished among five types of vertigo: those caused by body rotation, by galvanic (electrical) stimulation, by cerebral ischemia, by looking down from great heights, and from alcohol and other narcotics. Most of his experiments were on the first of these. He produced vertigo by rotating the body voluntarily, on a roundabout, and in a rotating chair. Initially he examined the introspective aspects of postrotary vertigo and made many experimental manipulations of it, as well as inducing vertigo by rotating the body in a specially designed chair. Purkinje described rotary and postrotary eye movements and suggested that "visual vertigo is a consequence of the conflict between unconscious involuntary muscular actions and voluntary conscious ones in the opposite direction" (1820, p. 95). In one characteristically heroic experiment he was rotated for 1 hr and then described the visual and somatosensory aftereffects that ensued! Among the few sources of earlier research he did cite was a translation of Erasmus Darwin's *Zoonomia* (Darwin, 1795) and Herz's (1786) medical text on dizziness and its treatment. Herz did refer to Willis' (1672) observations on body rotation and modified the interpretation slightly by referring to movement of nervous humors in the brain rather than the animal spirit.

Purkinje brought his ingenuity and insight to this topic, but he was lacking a thorough appreciation of the past work on it. Most particularly, he was unaware of similar, and in some respects more sophisticated, experiments that had been performed by Wells over 20 years earlier. Not only was Wells' (1792, 1794a, 1794b) work neglected by Purkinje himself, but those who have summarized Purkinje's work on vertigo (Bárány, 1913; Boring, 1942; Griffith, 1922; Grüsser, 1984; Kruta, 1964a) also failed to mention Wells. Dusser de Barenne (1934) did make passing reference to one of Wells' early observations, but failed to mention any of the afterimage experiments. Both Wells and Darwin had been stimulated to conduct their experiments on the basis of a report by Porterfield (1759). Purkinje (1825a) cited Porterfield in the *New Contributions*, but he was not referred to in the long articles of 1820 or 1827. It is unfortunate that Purkinje relied on Erasmus Darwin's treatment of vertigo because it was biased in several ways: Darwin refused to accept a link between eye movements and visual vertigo, and he denied the existence of ocular torsion.

Erasmus Darwin did, however, initiate studies that used devices to rotate the body, probably similar to those used later by Purkinje. In volume four of the third edition of *Zoonomia,* Darwin described a contraption he called a rotative couch. Although he provided a detailed illustration of it (made by his friend James Watt), he neither constructed one nor performed experiments with it. The intended purpose of the rotative couch was to increase pressure in the brain. Darwin described it thus (1801b):

> Another experiment I have frequently wished to try, which cannot be done in private practice, and which I therefore recommend to some hospital physician; and that is, to endeavour to still the violent actions of the heart and arteries, after due evacuations by venesection and cathartics, by gently compressing the brain. This might be done by suspending a bed, so as to whirl the patient round with his head most distant from the centre of rotation, as if he lay on a mill-stone.... For this purpose a perpendicular shaft armed with iron gudgeons might have one end pass into the floor, and the other into a beam in the ceiling, with a horizontal arm, to which a small bed may be readily suspended. By thus whirling the patient with increasing velocity sleep might be produced, and probably the violence of the actions of the heart and arteries might be diminished in inflammatory fevers.... What might be the consequence of whirling a person with his head next the centre of motion, so as to force the blood from the brain into the other parts of the body, might be discovered by cautious experiment without danger, and might probably add to our ability of curing fever. (pp. 436–438)

Darwin and Watt were members of the Lunar Society, which also included Matthew Boulton, Josiah Wedgwood, and Joseph Priestley (see King-Hele, 1977). Darwin's idea of passive body rotation was soon taken up by clinicians working in asylums for the insane. Cox (1804) was the first to construct and use Darwin's device, and he recommended the therapeutic effects of what was called swinging: "This is both a moral and a medical mean in the treatment of maniacs" (p. 102). He subjected the harnessed patients to either oscillatory motion, as on a conventional swing, or rotation in a chair or bed; the effects of body rotation were considered to be more efficacious than oscillation. Cox noted that "One of its most valuable properties is its proving a mechanical anodyne. After a few circumvolutions, I have witnessed the soothing lulling effects, when the mind has become tranquillized, and the body quiescent; a degree of vertigo has often followed, and this been succeeded by the most refreshing slumbers" (p. 104). Cox's book was translated into German, and the technique attracted widespread interest and application (see Grüsser, 1984). The technique was developed further by Hallaran (1818), who produced a linked system involving a chair and a bed that could be rotated at 100 rpm.

When Porterfield (1759) was conducting his studies he did not have the benefit of such controlled stimulation, and vertigo was induced in the time-honored manner of voluntary rotation of the upright body. He stated that the eyes did not move following rotation of the body, even though visual vertigo was pronounced. Despite objects' appearing to move in the direction opposite to prior rotation, the eyes were said to remain stationary: "If a Person turns swiftly round, without changing his Place, all Objects about will seem to move in a Circle to the contrary Way, and the Deception continues, not only when the Person himself moves round, but, which is more surprising, it also continues for some time after he stops moving, when the Eye, as well as the Objects, are at absolute Rest" (1759, p. 425). The phenomenon of visual vertigo following rotation had been described many times, but linking it with eye movements, or the absence of them, was novel. Porterfield was convinced, on the basis of his lack of any awareness, that his eyes did not move following rotation. The postrotary visual motion "proceeds from a Mistake we are in, with respect to the Eye; which, tho' it be absolutely at rest, we nevertheless conceive it as moving the contrary way to that in which it moved before: From which Mistake with respect to the Motion of the Eye, the Objects at rest will appear to move in the same way, which the Eye is imagined to move in, and consequently will seem to continue their Motion for some Time after the Eye is at rest" (p. 426). One reason for the widespread knowledge of Porterfield's observations was that his account was repeated almost verbatim by Priestley (1772) in his history of light and vision, which was soon translated into German (Priestley, 1776).

Robert Darwin (1786), the son of Erasmus and father of Charles, offered an alternative interpretation of postrotary apparent motion in an article on afterimages. He suggested that the sequence of light entering the eyes during rotation was visible as a moving afterimage when the body came to rest: "When any one turns round rapidly on one foot, till he becomes dizzy and falls upon the ground, the spectra of the ambient objects continue to present themselves in rotation, or appear to librate, and he seems to behold them for some time still in motion" (p. 315). The hypotheses of both Porterfield and Robert Darwin were roundly criticized by Wells (1792), who provided experimental evidence to refute them. The elegance of Wells' experiments lay not only in the description of the phenomenon but also in the use of afterimages, generated before rotation, to render visible the motions of the eyes after rotation ceased. Wells gave the first clear description of the fast and slow phases of postrotary nystagmus and its decreasing amplitude with time. Furthermore, he described how the direction of postrotary afterimage motion was the same as that of body rotation but the paper on which the afterimage was projected appeared to move in the opposite direction. The direction of visual motion following rotation was dependent on head position during rotation. Rotation with the head upright resulted in horizontal visual vertigo when the head remained upright, but when he tilted his head laterally to be horizontal the visual motion was vertical. Wells was not aware of feeling his eyes moving after rotation and so he asked another person to rotate and then stop "and I could plainly see, that, although he thought his eyes were fixed, they were in reality moving in their sockets, first toward one side, and then toward the other" (1792, p. 97). One of the few commentators to report on the studies by Porterfield and Wells on postrotary eye movements was Bell (1803). He concluded in Wells' favor with the following succinct statement: "How superior is simple experiment to the most ingenious speculation!" (p. 293).

Robert Darwin's article was reprinted as the final chapter in the first volume of Erasmus Darwin's *Zoonomia* in 1794. Indeed, Erasmus seems to have played more than a minor role in the writing of his son's paper, which was based on his doctoral dissertation in medicine (see King-Hele, 1999). Erasmus used large sections of Robert's article in other chapters of his book, particularly that on "The motions of the retina demonstrated by experiments," which was concerned with afterimages. A chapter on vertigo was included, but it was the "Additional observations on vertigo," which were appended to the reprint of Robert's article in which Erasmus supported his son's theory against the attack of Wells (see Cohen, 1984; Wade, 1998a, 2000c). Erasmus Darwin did not consider that eye movements were involved in postrotary visual motion for several reasons. First, he contended that visual motion continued for longer than eye movement. Second, he considered that the eyes rotated with equal velocity in both directions, and he did not distinguish between the slow and the fast phases of nystagmus. Third, he conducted an experiment (1794)

> in which the rolling of the eyes does not take place at all after revolving, and yet the vertigo is more distressing than in the situations above mentioned. If any one looks steadily at a spot in the ceiling over his head, or indeed at his own finger held up high over his head, and in that situation turns round till he becomes giddy; and then stops, and looks horizontally; he now finds, that the apparent rotation of objects is from above downwards, or from below upwards; that is, the apparent circulation of objects is now vertical instead of horizontal, making part of a circle round the axis of the eye; and this without any rolling of his eyeballs. The reason of there being no rolling of the eyeballs perceived after this experiment, is, because the images of objects are formed in rotation round the axis of the eye, and not from one side to the other of the axis of it; so that, as the eyeball has not the power to turn in its socket round its own axis, it cannot follow the apparent motions of these evanescent spectra, either before or after the body is at rest. (p. 572)

An additional factor was that giddiness could be experienced by a blind person; that is, Darwin confounded the visceral sensation of vertigo with its possible visual consequences. Accordingly, he dismissed the correlation between eye movements and visual motion for all forms of postrotary vertigo.

There followed two rejoinders by Wells (1794a, 1794b). First, he demonstrated that visual vertigo occurs with rotation in darkness, contrary to the Darwins' speculation. Second, he carried out experiments indicating not only that the eyes moved following body rotation (discounting Porterfield's position) but also how they moved. He provided, together with these, a phenomenological description of the reducing amplitude of postrotary nystagmus. Moreover, the apparent motion could be suppressed by fixation. Even more impressively, in the context of his dispute with Erasmus Darwin, Wells (1794b) demonstrated that the direction of nystagmus is dependent on the axis of the head during rotation and that torsional nystagmus followed rotating the upright body with the head tilted backward to view the ceiling.

Erasmus Darwin (1796) made some minor additions to his chapter on vertigo in the second edition of *Zoonomia*, and in volume one of the third edition (1801a) he returned to the issue of postrotary perception and briefly addressed Wells' objections. Darwin's views were modified slightly, but he remained convinced that visual vertigo was not associated with eye movements: "Whence I conclude, that vertigo may have for its cause either the ocular spectra of the sense of vision, when a person revolves with his eyes open; or the auricular murmurs of the sense of hearing, if he is revolved near a cascade; or the evanescent titillations of the sense of touch, if he revolves blindfold" (1801a, p. 346). In suggesting that bodily sensations generate visual vertigo in the last condition, Darwin failed to recognized the import of Wells' afterimage experiments.

Wells summarized his conclusions succinctly in his second retort: "When we stop ourselves while giddy from turning, our eyes do not return to the state of rest along with our bodies, but continue to move for some time after. Of this, however, we are not conscious; and hence we imagine the relative motion between our eyes and objects at rest to be possessed by the latter" (1794b, p. 905). Wells' experimental variations on this theme should be considered as laying the foundations for the study of visual–vestibular interaction that are usually attributed to Purkinje. It seems likely that Purkinje did not read English in the early part of his career and so would not have had access to Wells' book and articles. There was little in the translation of the first edition of Darwin's *Zoonomia* (1795) to suggest the subtlety of Wells' initial experiments in 1792.

Purkinje (1820) performed many of the experimental manipulations described by Wells and provided a general principle: "... the midpoint of the head (considered as a sphere), around which the first movement was performed, invariably determined the direction of apparent motion regardless of the subsequent position of the head" (p. 86). Kruta (1964a) referred to this as "Purkinje's law of vertigo." There was no clear indication of how such motions in the head could be detected, and his initial interpretation was conceptually little different from Willis' (1672) appeal to movements of the animal spirit: Purkinje suggested that, rather than the animal spirit showing inertia relative to the head, motion of the brain itself lagged behind that of the head, with particular influence exerted by the cerebellum. Purkinje concluded his first article with a statement that was soon to be realized: "It remains for a future work to establish the possible movements in the brain which measure its structure and organization" (1820, p. 125).

The significance of the vestibular system to the maintenance of posture and balance slowly emerged after Flourens (1824, 1830, 1842) conducted his lesion studies, initially on the cerebellum and later on the labyrinth of the inner ear. Marie Jean Pierre Flourens (1794–1867) was a harsh critic of Gall's (1822) phrenology, not so much in terms of its psychological speculations as its support of cortical localization. Flourens provided experimental evidence questioning functional localization in the brain. He was trained in medicine and became renowned for his skill as an experimental physiologist. The technique he introduced was that of extirpation or ablation: the surgical removal of parts of the brain to examine how the remainder functions by a study of postoperative behavior. His initial experiments examined extirpation of increasing parts of the cerebellum, said by Gall to be a center for amativeness or sexual responsiveness. The experimental animal (a dog) showed considerable impairment of motor control, but not of amativeness: "He had all his intellectual faculties, all his senses; he was only deprived of the faculty of coordinating and regularizing his movements" (Fancher, 1990, p. 82). Flourens' most productive period was in the 1820s with his experiments on reptiles, birds, and mammals, and he rarely made distinctions between the brains of these animals. His principal conclusions were these: "1. Despite the diversity of action of each of its parts, the whole nervous system is still a particular system; 2. Independently of the *proper action* of each part, each part has a *common action* with all the others, as have all the others with it" (Herrnstein & Boring, 1965, p. 223). Thus, he viewed the brain as having some degree of localized function, but that it acted as a unit. These ideas were to inhibit his association of the functions of the vestibular receptors with the control of equilibrium. In his experiments in the late 1820s he removed the semicircular canals of pigeons, and he was able to demonstrate that stimulation of a particular semicircular canal elicited nystagmus in the same plane as well as disturbances of posture and equilibrium: The body of the experimental animals always turned in the direction of the severed canal. Despite such strong experimental indications, the belief that the vestibular receptors were involved in hearing remained, and it was so cited by Müller in his *Handbuch* (see Müller, 1840, 1843). It was even suggested that the orientations of the semicircular canals served the function of locating the direction of sound.

Purkinje (1826, 1827a) saw the relevance of Flourens' experiments to his own studies of vertigo, and he was impressed by the selective disturbances of motor coordination produced by cerebellar lesions. These led to a change in his interpretation of vertigo: rather than considering that the brain as a whole moved, rather like Willis' fluid in a flask, he attributed the effects to movements associated with the cerebellum. He stated that "the cerebellum is the seat of the spatial sense" (1826, p. 120), but the manner in which it operated remained a mystery.

The mode of signaling accelerations of the head by inertial motion of the endolymph in the semicircular canals was described independently by Mach, Breuer, and Crum Brown in the early 1870s (see Henn, 1984; Howard & Templeton, 1966). During head rotation the endolymph in the canals displaces receptors in the ampulla, signaling angular accelerations and exerting control over posture and eye movements. At last there was a theory that was free from the influence of animal spirit, although the proposed motion of the endolymph in the canals was remarkably similar to the fluid analogies made by Willis (1672). Alexander Crum Brown (1874, 1875) based his analysis on thresholds for detecting body rotation on a revolving stool; the thresholds were lowest when the head was positioned so that one of the semicircular canals was in the plane of rotation. Ernst Mach (1873, 1875) constructed a rotating chair that was mounted in a rotatable frame. He examined the perception of the visual vertical during static tilt and also the visual aftereffects of body rotation. From such experiments with this apparatus he concluded that "one therefore does not sense angular velocity, but rather angular acceleration" (Henn, 1984, p. 146). Mach made the explicit connection between Purkinje's experiments on vertigo and the function of the semicircular canals. Josef Breuer (1874) followed in the tradition of Flourens by making systematic lesions of the semicircular canals of pigeons. Breuer also distinguished between the canal receptors and the otolith organs of the vestibular system, which detected orientation with respect to gravity.

Long before these developments, Wells was aware, on theoretical grounds, that there must be some system that registers the position of the body with respect to gravity: "In the estimates we make by sight of the situation of external objects, we have always some secret reference to the position of our own bodies, with respect to the plane of the horizon" (1792, p. 85). Although he asked "What is there within us, to indicate these positions of the body?" (p. 86) he could not answer to his satisfaction, as he could only draw on the actions of the voluntary muscles. However, he did refrain from an appeal to motion of the animal spirit in the head.

Following his long article in 1820, Purkinje returned to the issue of vertigo in a number of briefer reports and reviews, as well as in the *New Contributions*; some of the articles were later assembled as an appendix to Aubert (1888) and all are in volumes 2, 3, and 5 of Purkinje's *Opera Omnia*. Purkinje's active experimentation on vertigo ceased before he had been able to integrate adequately the later lesion studies of Flourens (see Kruta, 1964a). It was not until Flourens described experiments specifically sectioning the semicircular canals (in 1828) that the link between their function and vertigo was potentially apparent, although Flourens himself did not draw the parallels (see McKendrick & Gray, 1900), nor was the hydrodynamic theory proposed until much later in the century.

NEUROSCIENCE

The light cast at the commencement of neuroscience was not generated by any single individual alone. The endeavors of many conspired to illuminate the structure of the nervous system, the manner of electrical communication within it, its links to reflexes and to more complex behavior, as well as to perceptual experience. Of course, neuroscience itself did not exist in the early 19th century. It is a neologism of recent years and was defined by Thompson (1986) in terms of the activities practiced by its adherents: "Neuroscientists study all aspects of the brain, its structure and development, the chemical and electrical phenomena occurring in its neurons and how these interact, and the brain's unique output, behavior and experience. The nervous system, particularly its anatomy and elementary functions, has been studied for centuries, but the field of neuroscience as a unified discipline is only a few years old" (p. vii).

Many of the phenomena mentioned above, as well as those in chapters 3 and 4, remain at the center of neuroscience. They provide examples of Purkinje's desire for exact subjectivism—to provide physiological accounts of subjective experiences. At that time there was a much longer history of describing experiences rather than physiology, and so the physiological accounts that could be given were indeed elementary. Nonetheless, embarking on the enterprise was itself worthy of note. One of the phenomena mentioned above—the motion aftereffect—features prominently in contemporary neuroscience; the whole armory of recording and brain imaging devices has been trained on finding correlates of the experience of motion when one is viewing stationary objects (see Mather, et al., 1998).

The claim that Purkinje witnessed the dawning of neuroscience does not depend on his exact subjectivism alone. Neuroscience has emerged from the biological sciences because the conceptual building blocks have been isolated, and the ways in which they can be arranged are being explored. Purkinje was partially responsible for fashioning the two foundations on which the structure could be securely built: the cell and the neuron doctrines. The emergence of both doctrines was dependent on the development of achromatic microscopes and microtomes so that the sections of anatomical specimens could be examined in greater detail.

Cells were described soon after the first microscopes were focused on animal matter. Robert Hooke (1665) gave them the name "cells," and he identified plant cells. A variety of animal cells, including nerve fibers, was described by Antonius van Leeuwenhoek (1674, 1675). The microscopic world was transformed by the introduction of powerful achromatic instruments in the 1830s, and rapid advances were made thereafter. The cell doctrine was most clearly articulated at the end of that decade by Theodor Schwann: "There is one common principle of development for the most diverse elementary parts of the organism, and that this principle is the formation of cells" (1839, p. 196).

Purkinje obtained a Plössl microscope in 1832 and, together with his students (most notably Gabriel Valentin), examined a wide range of structures. In a letter to one of his students he wrote that "There should be nothing in the whole organic body that cannot be investigated and identified with regard to its detail and its local and general function" (Thomsen, 1919, p. 1). The cerebellum was one of the structures examined. Purkinje described the microscopic characteristics of the large cells in the "yellow" (white) matter on 23 September 1837 to a meeting of natural scientists held in Prague:

> Similar corpuscles are present everywhere in the folia of the cerebellum, arranged in great numbers in rows delimiting the yellow matter. Each of these corpuscles is turned with its rounded end inward, towards the yellow matter, and in its head, apart from the inner space, there is also distinctly shown a central nucleus. Its tail is turned outward and, mostly ending in two projections, buries itself in the grey matter almost as far as the outer periphery, where the surface is surrounded by the vascular membrane. (Kruta, 1971, p. 127)

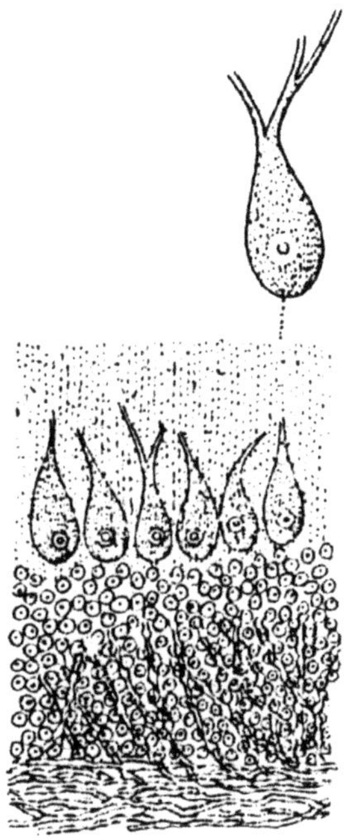

FIG. 1.3. Purkinje cells. Purkinje's (1837a) diagram of cells in the cerebellum.

A diagram of what are now called Purkinje cells is shown in Fig. 1.3. An earlier illustration was provided by Valentin (1836), who stated that "This observation was first made by Purkyně in sheep, and I succeeded later in finding the same structure in man, the calf, the pig, and the horse, at this site as well as in the yellow substance of the cerebral hemispheres" (Clarke & O'Malley, 1968, p. 45). In summarizing these early investigations, Liddell (1960) concluded that "To Purkinje therefore goes credit for the first clear account of nerve cells and the processes of nerve cells in the brain and spinal cord, as well as confirming with the new microscope that nerve tubes contained marrow. Schwann's 'cell theory' came in 1839, but Purkinje had discerned the true state of affairs some two years before Schwann" (p. 8).

These observations were made before any adequate staining methods had been developed. Purkinje used alcohol to fix his preparations, and he made thin sections so that they could be examined microscopically. Kruta (1971) noted that "Purkyně was one of the first—at least after Leewenhoek—to observe tissues in thin sections and he thus contributed considerably to the improvement of microscopic technique" (p. 127). The staining procedures introduced later in the 19th century verified the speculations about the continuity between nerve cells and their fibers but they did not clarify the anatomical relationship among the nerves themselves. There were two opposing camps: On the one hand, the reticularists argued that all nerves were linked continuously in a vast network; the anti-reticularists, on the other hand, believed that neurons were structurally independent units of nervous activity. It was not until the end of the century that the neuron doctrine was finally accepted. It was firmly established by evidence about the synapse, the term introduced by Sherrington, who proposed a mode of chemical transmission across the synaptic junctions. The fascinating history of this period has been variously chronicled by Brazier (1988), Clarke and O'Malley (1968), Finger (1994), Liddell (1960), McHenry (1969), Rose and Bynum (1982), Shepherd (1991), Spillane (1981), and Wade (2000d).

Purkinje was not only a pioneer of perception but also of neuropharmacology. As a medical student he spent much time learning to distinguish among different drugs by taste and smell, and he conducted experiments on the effects of self-administered drugs. Writing later in his life, he noted: "From the beginning of my medical studies I was mainly interested in physiology. It seemed to me to be very important and interesting to learn the effects of drugs on the healthy organism. I considered this study as a substantial part of physiology as a whole where little had been done.... The original idea, i.e. the need for physiological examination of drugs, sank deep into my memory and I tried to test some drugs on my own body" (Votava, 1971, p. 48). Among those Purkinje tested were ipecacuanha, digitalis, opium, belladonna, stramonium, turpentine, camphor, and nutmeg. He gave himself measured doses and recorded the consequences for his general mental state. The effects of belladonna on accommodation have been discussed above. Votava remarked "he was not only a pioneer in the field of drug self-experimentation, but also a hero among scientists" (1971, p. 55).

PSYCHOLOGY

Neuroscience is a multidisciplinary endeavor in much the same way that Purkinje envisaged the physiology of his day. He considered that "the physiologist must be a chemist, a physicist, and a psychologist" (Brožek & Hoskovec, 1987, p. 14), reflecting the influence of *Naturphilosophie* on his outlook. Thus the scope of Purkinje's purview of physiology was truly remarkable, and it took in psychology, too. He was first and foremost a physiologist, but the line dividing physiology from psychology at the beginning of the 19th century was a thin one, particularly in the province of the senses (see Hatfield, 1990). His exact subjectivism would place him in the mainstream of contemporary perceptual psychology. He intentionally included the term subjective or introspective (*heautognostisch*) in his early publications, but he did not wish his interpretations to be restricted to that level alone.

There exist two other sources that reflect his concerns with psychology—his lecture notes on empirical psychology and on physiological psychology, and a series of "psychological fragments"— that have been assembled by Brožek and Hoskovec (1987). The lecture notes were in German and the fragments in Czech, and they provide valuable insights into Purkinje's approaches to the senses, psychology, and science. The lecture notes relate to his tenure in Breslau (1823–1850), and the lectures were delivered throughout the fertile period of his microscopic studies in the 1830s. The psychological fragments were probably written in the 1860s.

The definitions Purkinje gave of psychology reflect the lingering influence of German romantic physiology, as Rothschuh (1973) has called it, by embracing an interplay between the rational and the empirical. His influences were from not only German thinkers like Kant, Schelling, Goethe, and Fichte, but also from the British empiricists, Locke, Berkeley, Hume, and Reid. Berkeley, in particular, was singled out as providing the appropriate combination of idealism and empiricism; he is referred to by Purkinje as "the originator of empirical psychology." Purkinje's studies of the senses epitomize this contrast; introspective descriptions are subjected to physiological interpretations. Many of the psychological dimensions listed involve contrasting pairs: "In every single class of experience one finds conditions of positive and negative contrasts.... There are many contrasts in the sphere of the senses.... Blue and yellow, red and green" (Brožek & Hoskovec, 1987, p. 55). Could this be the embryo of Hering's opponent process of color vision? Purkinje acknowledged that a rigorous empirical psychology was still lacking at that time, although he foresaw it as one based on physiology.

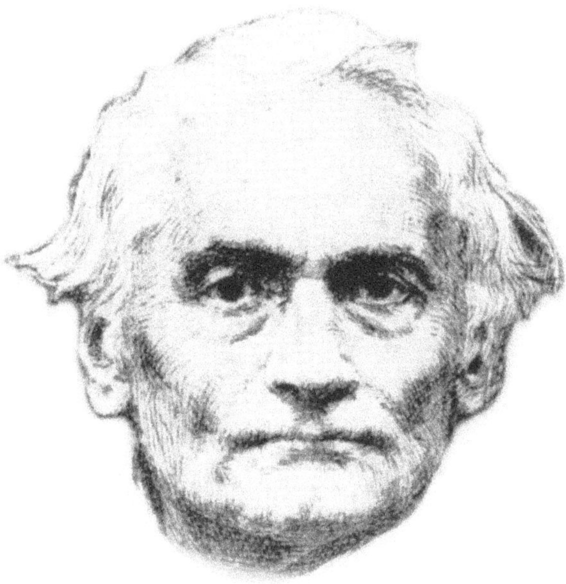

FIG. 1.4. Portrait of Purkinje after an illustration in Psotníčková (1955).

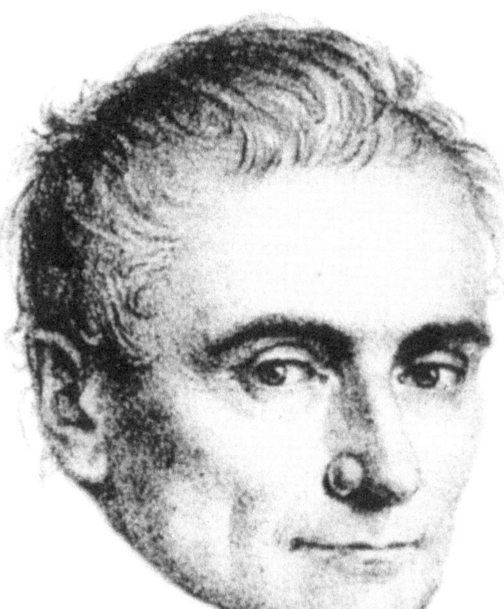

FIG. 2.1. Portrait of Purkinje after a frontispiece illustration in *Opera Omnia*, volume 3.

2

Biographical and Bibliographical Notes

EARLY LIFE

Jan Evangelista Purkinje was born on 17 December 1787 in the town of Libochovice in the north of Bohemia and died on 28 July 1868 in Prague. He was the first son of Josef Purkinje, who served as economic supervisor of the holdings of the family Dietrichstein, and Rosalie, born Safranek. He had a happy childhood until 1793, when his father died suddenly. This profoundly affected the economic status of the family, and Jan's opportunity to acquire higher education was endangered (see Kotek and Niklicek, 1987).

Jan received the foundations of general education in the Czech primary school of his birthplace. The inquisitive child widened his horizons by reading Comenius' *Orbis Pictus* (*The World in Pictures*). The local chaplain was impressed by the child's intelligence and introduced him to Latin. He also taught him the Greek alphabet and spoke with him about astronomy. In the school Jan was introduced to music, both vocal and instrumental. He sang well and learned to play violin. As it turned out, these skills, especially singing, were of critical importance for the continuation of his education.

In the spring of 1798, with the help of his mother's friends, Jan was accepted as a member of the church choir in Mikulov, in southern Moravia. This enabled him to attend the school, established for the Piarist order by Cardinal Dietrichstein, without paying the relatively high tuition fees. The language of instruction was German. The study program involved 3 years of the so-called normal school and 5-year gymnasium. At the gymnasium, the curriculum included Latin, Greek, history, and geography. In contrast to other comparable schools, at this gymnasium the Piarists paid substantial attention to philosophy, modern languages, mathematics, and physics. The Mikulov school had a rich collection of astronomical and physical apparatus.

Jan did well in the normal school and was one of the best students at the gymnasium; he completed his studies there in 1804. In order to be able to continue his schooling, he applied for admission to the Piarist order and was accepted. For his novitiate he journeyed to the monastery Stara Voda (Old Water), near Olomouc, in north–central Moravia. Here he strengthened his knowledge of some subjects that were taught in the gymnasium and also learned French and Italian.

In 1805 Purkinje began to teach at the Piarist school at Straznice, in southern Moravia, and in the following year he moved to the Piarist college in Litomysl, in eastern Bohemia. During the school year 1806–1807 he simultaneously taught at the normal school and studied philosophy; the latter was at a school training future gymnasium teachers as well as students planning to study law, medicine, or theology.

The library of the monastery of Olomouc offered rich treasures. Among the major German thinkers, Kant remained unappealing to Purkinje whereas Schelling's *Naturphilosophie* (*Philosophy of Nature*) interested him throughout his life. However, it was Fichte who affected him most profoundly, especially through "Some lectures on the mission of a scholar" (Einige Vorlesungen über die Bestimmung des Gelehrten, 1794) and "The call of men to an unlimited mental freedom" (Über die Bestimmung des Menschen zur unbeschränkten seelischen Freiheit, 1800).

The German philosophers were not the most appropriate reading matter for a thoughtful young cleric who was a member in the Piarist order. Purkinje himself, in his midseventies, remembered the impact of Fichte's philosophy as follows: "Having become somewhat familiar with the state of the newer literature in Germany and in other cultured countries and admiring their top contributors as well as getting to know the fate of my aging colleagues in the monastery, exhausted from an early age by strenuous teaching, I was frightened that a similar fate would await me as well" (Rieger, 1867, p. 1115). Fichte's philosophy vividly portrayed the mission of a true scholar in human society and rallied the human mind to an unlimited freedom. In combination with this familiarity with Fichte, Purkinje began to think of a different, happier life with enough strength to establish an independent position in the world: "Yes, the desire of glory strongly impelled me to follow my own path. Having been concerned in the monastery only with philological and historical studies, I turned first to poetry and then to philosophy whose spirit would free my mind. Yes, I felt deeply that I could achieve something significant in natural sciences, about which of course I had only a vague idea" (Rieger, 1867, p. 1115). These thoughts moved Purkinje to leave the Piarist order. The chronicle of the monastery at Litomysl contains a brief record of his decision: *Clericus Silverius Purkinie deserto Instituto nostro ad parentes Libochovicium migravit* ("Having left our institution, the Clericus Silverius [his Piarist name] moved to his parents in Libochovice").

In the years 1807–1809 Purkinje studied in the second and the third years of the philosophical faculty of the University of Prague, then known as "Universitas Carolo—Ferdinandea." His interests were turning more and more toward the natural sciences. In his old age he noted that physics was his first love. In the second year he completed a manuscript on Chladni's sound images and handed it into his professor of physics, F. Schmidt, who was director of the Physical Institute of the Faculty of Philosophy. Purkinje returned to the subject more than 10 years later. Among the teachers of the faculty of philosophy, the botanist and mineralogist Jan Emanuel Pohl, an adherent of *Naturphilosophie*, had the most influence on him. Having finished studies at the Faculty of Philosophy, Purkinje found himself lacking the means for continuing his studies. In 1809 Pohl recommended Purkinje as tutor to the son of the Baron Franz Hildprandt, owner of properties in Blatna in the southwestern part of Bohemia. At Blatna Purkinje spent three rewarding years in a cultured environment and with possibilities of studying in the rich library of the castle.

The ideas of Novalis and the writing of the Swiss pedagogue Pestalozzi stimulated Purkinje's interest in institutions in which children were to be educated by outstanding teachers, without the "disturbing impact of the families." In fact, at Blatna he played with the idea of creating just such an institution. As Purkinje later recalled, in such an institution the children would receive multifaceted training, including handicrafts, trades, and arts, but also experimentation and the use of instruments. Their physical, intellectual, emotional, and motivational development would be influenced in practical ways, as specified by Pestalozzi (see Rieger, 1867). Purkinje did not pursue the idea of such a career. Thanks to the financial assistance provided by his former employer, in November 1812, Purkinje was able to enter the medical faculty of the University of Prague.

The medical faculty operated at a contemporary international level of natural and medical sciences. Prominent among his teachers were the anatomist Johann Georg Ilg, physiologist and ophthalmologist Josef Rottenberger, and Andreas Wawruch, a pathologist and teacher of *materia medica*, the science dealing with the nature and properties of substances used in treating diseases. Ilg was a believer in empirical knowledge in contrast to speculations, and he taught anatomy with his own textbook, *Grundlinien der Zergliederungskunde des menschlichen Körpers* (1811), published at the very start of his teaching at the medical faculty of Prague. He was well known for his skillful autopsies and for preparation of anatomical teaching specimens. Rottenberger lectured on physiology and, more importantly for Purkinje's scientific career, ophthalmology. These lectures contributed to the Purkinje's choice of vision as the topic of his doctoral dissertation (Rieger, 1867). Another important factor for Purkinje's professional career was his contact with I. Fritz, a skillful and original surgeon. Purkinje learned from him basic operational techniques, but also gained his personal friendship. Fritz supported Purkinje's subsequent search for employment that would permit him to put to use and further develop his talent for scientific research. The lectures of Wawruch on *materia medica* inspired Purkinje to examine the impact of some medicaments on himself (Kotek and Niklicek, 1987)

It was in 1818 that Fritz and Wawruch brought Purkinje to the attention of the Professor of Surgery, J. V. Rust, in Berlin. Rust supported the nomination of Purkinje for a Prussian travel fellowship, with the prospect of a professorship in veterinary science. Purkinje did not accept the offer, as he decided, at Hildprandt's suggestion, to complete his medical studies by defending a doctoral dissertation. Nevertheless, he acquired in Rust a significant protector.

Purkinje's defense of his doctoral dissertation, "Beiträge zur Kenntniss des Sehens in subjektiver Hinsicht" (Contribution to the Knowledge of Vision in its Subjective Aspects), took place on 30 November 1818. The notice announcing the defense is shown in Fig. 2.2, together with the title page of his candidate's dissertation. The dissertation appeared in print in Prague in 1819 and again in 1823, and a translation is given in chapter 4.

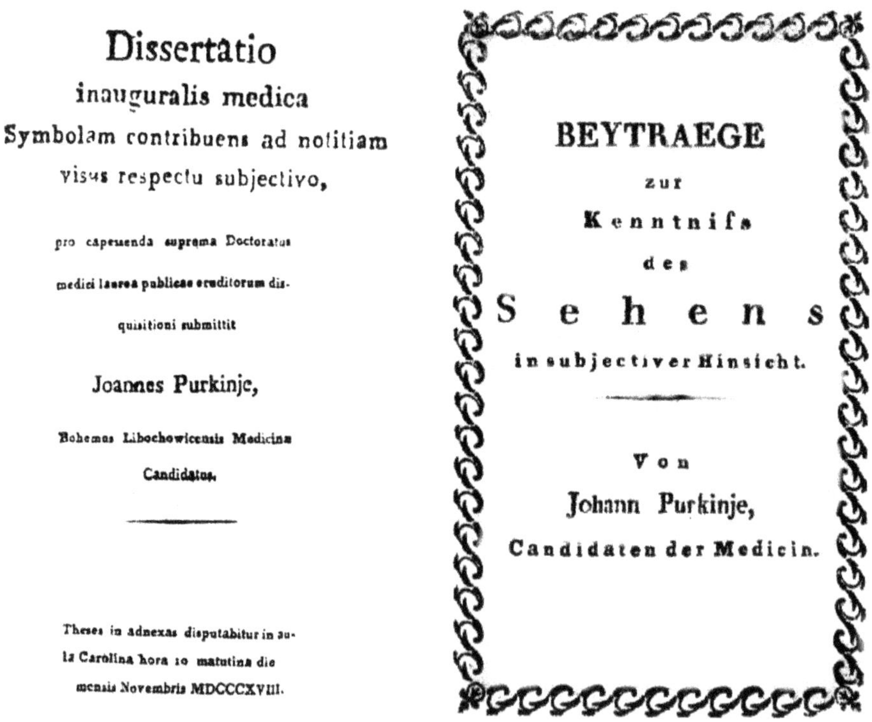
Dissertatio
inauguralis medica
Symbolam contribuens ad notitiam
visus respectu subjectivo,
pro capessenda suprema Doctoratus
medici laurea publicae eruditorum disquisitioni submittit
Joannes Purkinje,
Bohemus Libochowicensis Medicinae
Candidatus.
Theses in adnexas disputabitur in aula Carolina hora 10 matutina die
mensis Novembris MDCCCXVIII.

BEYTRAEGE
zur
Kenntniſs
des
Sehens
in subjectiver Hinsicht.
Von
Johann Purkinje,
Candidaten der Medicin.

FIG. 2.2. Notice announcing the defense of Purkinje's doctoral dissertation and the title page of the unpublished dissertation (from Psotníčková, 1955).

PURKINJE'S VIEWS OF PSYCHOLOGY

Toward the end of his life, Purkinje recalled, with amusement, his early fascination with faculty psychology: "Just prior to and following Kant, a terminology operating with abstract concepts came into vogue as an odd mythology. All mental activities and faculties that could possibly be differentiated received separate names and were placed in proper ranks like the gods on Mount Olympus. Imagination, feeling, and desire led the chorus, with the minor gods following at proper distancies. What a striking picture of a large, colorful family!" (Brožek & Hoskovec, 1987, p. 117). It appears that Wetzel (1800, 1805), using this approach, reached the pinnacle in anthropological psychology, consisting of two thick volumes. In 1806, while Purkinje was studying Wetzel's book in the solitude of a monastery, he made for himself a detailed listing of all the mental faculties and powers, using a large sheet of paper meant for the writing of music. He thought that he had captured this elusive Proteus.

To Purkinje, psychology was an essential part of the complex of physiological sciences (*Cyklus der physiologischen Doktrinen*). In his review of Burdach's textbook of *Physiology as an Empirical Science*, Purkinje wrote in 1833 that "Mathematics, physics . . . but also chemistry, morphology and psychology . . . are essential parts of physiology." Years later Purkinje returned to the subject in his volume entitled *Academia*, published in 1861, and intended as a design for the Czech National Academy of Sciences. Purkinje wrote: "Physiology studies life phenomena in their chemical, physical, but also dynamic and psychological aspects. Since it is difficult, if not impossible for one man to master chemistry, physics and psychology, it will be necessary to employ in the institute specialists who will be concerned with each of these fields."

Purkinje returned to the nature of psychology in a fragment, written in Czech, toward the end of his life. "So far psychology had been viewed as a part of philosophy. Each new (philosophical) system came up with a new psychology. Only recently Herbart and his followers treated psychology as an empirical science" (Brožek & Hoskovec, 1987, p. 114). Then he continued "However, a rigorously empirical psychology does not yet exist. It can be developed only by a physiological approach. This involves comparing the results of introspective data with material phenomena. The beginnings have been made by men like K. Ph. Moritz, J. Müller, R. H. Lotze, A. Quetelet, M. J. P. Flourens. We can expect much from the newer neurology" (Brožek & Hoskovec, 1987, p. 116).

PSYCHOLOGICAL CONTRIBUTIONS DURING THE BRESLAU YEARS

The years spent in Breslau (1823–1850) were remarkably productive, with the principal focus on microscopic morphology. Here we note developments relevant to psychology. The first two years yielded two additional publications concerned with vision. The text of Purkinje's inaugural address, entitled *Physiological Examination of the Organ of Vision*, was presented on 22 December 1823 at the University of Vratislavia (Breslau), and reprinted in 1918 in Purkinje's *Opera Omnia*. A Czech version was prepared by the editor of volume 1 of Purkinje's *Opera Omnia*, Lhotak. In turn, H. J. John translated the Czech version into English (John, 1959). The English translation was published in volume 49 of the *Memoirs of the American Philosophical Society* and reprinted in Sahakian's *History of Psychology* (1968, pp. 101–108). The text deals with such topics as accommodation, effects of color and intensity illumination, ability of the eye to follow moving objects, direct and indirect vision, and location of the optic nerve into the retina.

In 1825 Purkinje published his *Neue Beiträge zur Kenntniss des Sehens in subjectiver Hinsicht* (*New Contributions to the Knowledge of Vision in its Subjective Aspects)* (1825a).

The volume contains 18 chapters. Their titles are as follows:

1. Indirect Vision
2. Galvanic Light Figures
3. Real and Apparent Movements
4. Elliptical Light Streaks
5. Faint Elliptical Area Produced by Contraction and Sudden Relaxation of Eyelids
6. A Field of Hazy Patches
7. Automatic Continuous Generation of Light in a Darkened Visual Field
8. Spider Web Figure
9. Sleepiness of the Eyes
10. Investigations of the Interaction of Colors
11. On Pressure Figures
12. A Shadowy Circle in the Middle of the Visual Field
13. Additional Methods for Making Visible the Veins of the Retina
14. Focal Image Inside the Eye
15. On Flicker in Front of the Eyes after the Use of Digitalis
16. Some Comments on Distance and Near Vision
17. Intentional Squinting
18. Effect of Belladonna on Vision

The description of the Purkinje shift was in chapter 10, as was outlined in the previous chapter.

Purkinje intended to publish, in addition to his two *Contributions*, two other volumes dealing with the senses. The third volume was to contain additional material dealing with vision; the fourth volume was to deal with other senses. Actually, a substantial amount of the material was ready for publication. There were two reasons for delaying the completion of the third volume of *Contributions*. First, Tourtual (1827) published a volume on *Human Senses with Reference to*

Mutual Relations of Psychological and Organic Processes. Purkinje emphasized that Tourtual's approach to the study of visual phenomena was very close to his own. The second, and probably more important, reason was that Purkinje's interests shifted to the study of anatomical and microscopical issues. Nevertheless, he hoped that he would be able to return to psychological studies. The fact that he did return is documented by two fragments, written in Czech in 1857, dealing with space perception.

During the years spent at the medical school at Breslau, Purkinje offered courses on psychology. These lectures were registered in the university catalogues, published both in Latin (*Indices Lectionum in Viadrina Vratislaviense*) and in German (*Vorlesungs—Verzeichnisse Universitaet Breslau*). All of Purkinje's lectures in psychology were given in the summer semesters. The lectures were offered first *privatim* and then *publice*. For those on empirical psychology offered privately, the students had to receive the professor's prior approval; the lecture given "publically" did not require such an approval. The lectures on empirical psychology were presented in 1827 and 1836; the lectures on physiological psychology were given in 1840 and 1842. The texts of the lecture notes were written in a not easily readable German script. The original manuscripts are held in Prague in the Literary Archives of the Museum of Czech Literature. The texts of the lecture notes have been transcribed and published (Brožek and Hoskovec, 1987, pp. 20–99). Their context and significance were the subject of a separate paper (Brožek and Hoskovec, 1988), accompanied by a summary in Russian and in English. The significance of Purkinje's lecture notes may be viewed from a biographical and from a scientific point of view. Biographically their significance is substantial: They document that Purkinje's interests and activities involved not only research, but also the teaching of psychology. Scientifically, the lecture notes are for the most part disappointing.

Purkinje's Breslau period was one of acute observation. In the first phase, up to about 1832, his vision was applied naturally; thereafter he was assisted by one of Plössl's achromatic microscopes to observe a new and relatively undistorted world of cells. Purkinje was also innovative in establishing a physiological laboratory in which students were actively engaged in experimental work. It is believed to have been one of the first such independent institutes (see Rothschuh, 1973). The early years in Breslau were personally fruitful for Purkinje. In 1827 he married Julia Rudolphi, the daughter of Karl A. Rudophi, Professor of Anatomy and Physiology at Berlin. The Purkinje's had two sons, but Julia died in 1835.

OBJECTIVE PSYCHOLOGY

The history of the term objective psychology is complex (Brožek, 1971, 1989, 1990). It is not clear who coined the term. Furthermore it may have occurred on more than one occasion. There is evidence that it was used by Purkinje in his lectures on empirical psychology offered during the summer semester of 1827.

The relevant passage, translated from the German original (Brožek and Hoskovec, 1987, p. 21) reads as follows: "In gathering psychological data we begin by bringing to mind a variety of facts that we experienced, beginning in our own childhood, the information is supplemented and organized. In addition, new data are generated in the course of psychological experiments. In this way it becomes possible to characterize our mental life in a general way. The study of the more specific mental phenomena leads us beyond ourselves into the human society (so that we can examine the individual differences in intellect and emotions), into the realm of history and the world of poetry, and finally into nature (in which we can study animal instincts and drives). Consequently, we can differentiate between a subjective psychology (self-knowledge, Autognosie) and an objective psychology."

During his stay in Breslau Purkinje published some psychological articles in Czech, including accounts on visual space (Purkinje, 1837c, 1840). In German, Purkinje (1846a) contributed a substantial entry on "senses in general" to the *Handwörterbuch der Physiologie* (*Dictionary of Physiology*). An extensive account on "wakefulness, sleep, dreams and related states" is also published in Wagner's *Handwörterbuch* (Purkinje, 1846b).

RETURN TO PRAGUE

Following the death of his wife and several close friends Purkinje felt more and more isolated in Breslau and yearned to return to Prague. Finally, he received a call to a chair of physiology at the University. He returned permanently to Prague on 9 April 1850. Purkinje's address was given on the occasion of the opening of the Physiological Institute of the University of Prague on 6 October 1851, and it concerned the relation of physiology to sciences and arts and the methods of its theoretical and practical study. It appeared both in Czech (Purkinje, 1851) and in German (Purkinje, 1852). Several publications, in Czech, are concerned with psychological topics. They include an article on the senses in general (1853a) and on the topology of the senses (1853b); the latter article appeared in German as well (Purkinje, 1854).

In 1857, three publications, written in Czech, were concerned with sleep and wakefulness. They dealt with wakefulness, its degrees, and the passage into degrees of sleep (1857a), the phenomena of sleep in the human and animal realm (1857b), and the physiology of sleep (1857c). An extensive account of Purkinje's older and newer publications appeared in the same year (1857d) and was continued in the next year (1858). An assessment of Purkinje's investigation in vision appeared in German in 1860, and an extensive account, in four installments, was published in 1864/65 and in 1865/66 (in Czech).

In 1867, shortly before his death, Purkinje published in both Czech and German a volume entitled *Austria Polyglotta*—a kind of applied social psychology, advocating a wider learning of the languages of nations comprising the Austrian empire as means for facilitating their peaceful coexistence.

ADDITIONAL CONTRIBUTIONS

References to conditioned responses, both muscular and visceral, can be found in Purkinje's early writings. In chapter 18 of his dissertation (1819/1823a), entitled "Voluntary Movements of the Pupil," the pupil was observed to widen when the subject focused on a more distant point and narrow down when a nearer point was focused. Eventually a representation (image) of one or other stimulus sufficed to generate the pupillomotor response. The relevant chapter was translated into Czech by Dostalek (1976, p. 23). In 1820 Purkinje reported observations on the formation of conditioned visceral responses in connection with his studies on the effects of emetine. Specifically, he observed the formation of a conditioned sensation of nausea to the color of emetine (an alkaloid obtained from ipecac) (Brožek, 1973). Later (Purkinje, 1857d), in reviewing in Czech his older investigations, Purkinje wrote the following: "I have reported an idiosyncratic response I acquired during experiments with emetine and which lasted for several days. Everytime I saw a brown color, similar to the color of emetine, I have experienced a sensation of nausea." Purkinje did not report that the phenomenon had been described by Whytt (1763).

Purkinje was an avid reader and a diligent reviewer of books. The book reviews relevant to psychology include the works of Johannes Müller (Purkinje, 1827b), Tourtual (Purkinje 1828a), and Ehrenberg (Purkinje, 1837b). He also wrote a note on Berkeley's contributions to the theory of vision (Purkinje, 1828b). A larger handwritten statement was to serve as introduction to a series of Purkinje's brief communications that were to be published under the title *Psychological Fragments*. The original text, in Czech, handwritten in the 1860s, was included in a volume entitled *J. E. Purkinje and Psychology, with a Focus on Unpublished Manuscripts* (Brožek & Hoskovec, 1987, pp. 114–116), which was followed by a translation into English entitled *A Glance at Contemporary Psychology* (pp. 116–118). In turn, the translation was reprinted in the *History of Psychology Newsletter* of the American Psychological Association (Brožek, 1988).

OPERA OMNIA

Purkinje's collected works (*Opera Omnia*) have been published in 13 volumes that spanned almost 70 years (1918–1985). They are not assembled in chronological sequence, but all the works by him cited here are printed in the volumes. A single volume of selected works (*Opera Selecta*) has also been published (Purkinje, 1948), and it contains his most influential publications; these include his doctoral dissertation, his inaugural lecture at Breslau, the description of the germinal vesicle in the egg yolk, reports on cell histology to the Society of German natural scientists, as well as other publications on cellular structure.

The two books on subjective visual phenomena (Purkinje 1823a, 1825a) are reprinted in first volume of the *Opera Omnia*, together with the *Commentatio* (1823b), the second edition of *Symbolae ad Ovi Avium* (1830), and the monograph

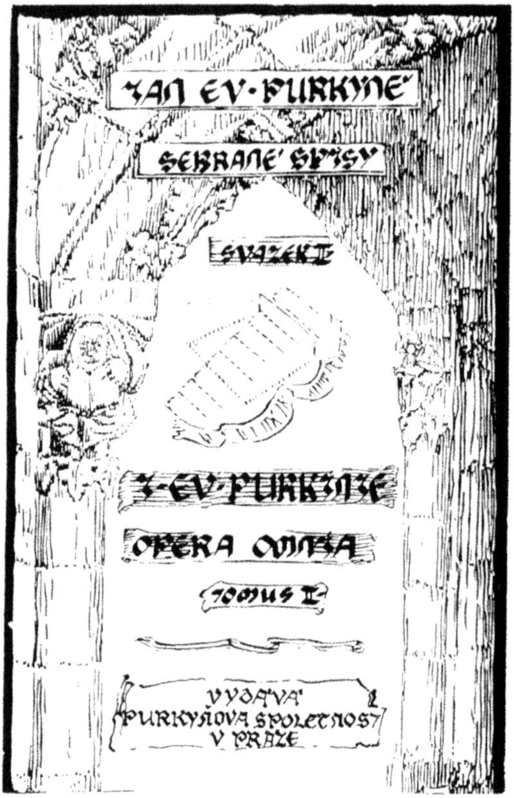

FIG. 2.3. Title page of *Opera Omnia*, volume 2.

on ciliary motion. Many of the short articles Purkinje published during his years in Breslau comprise the main contents of volume 2 (see Fig. 2.3). Several short pieces on subjective visual phenomena, published in the early 1820s, were assembled to form the substance of the second *Neue Beiträge* of 1825. There is also the long article on vertigo of 1820, as well as several shorter reports essentially repeating the descriptions of the phenomena. Most of the articles are reprinted from the natural science section of the *Schlesischen Gesellschaft für vaterländische Kultur*, and they cover an enormously broad range of topics—from histology to the reform of the secondary educational system!

Volume 3 assembles the reports of conference presentations, principally on cell structure. There is also Purkinje's (1827a) article on vertigo, integrating Flourens' studies with the lesion experiments of his student, Krauss, and with the earlier subjective reports of vertigo. The three chapters in Wagner's *Handwörterbuch* (on microscopes, the senses, and sleep) are reprinted in this volume. Purkinje contributed over 40 entries to the *Encyclopädisches Wörterbuch der medicinischen*

Wissenschaften for the volumes published between 1828 and 1834, and these are the main contents of volume 4. Purkinje's father-in-law, Rudolphi, was one of the editors of the encyclopedia. The topics ranged from *Achromatopsia* to *Erzeugung*, and included association, consciousness, cranioscopy, digestion, and elasticity. Vertigo is returned to in volume 5. Purkinje's (1826) review of Flourens' (1824) book is reprinted, as are the reviews of Müller's two books of 1826 (Müller, 1826a, 1826b), Burdach's (1819–1826) books on the brain, and Tortual's (1827) survey of the senses. Reviews of literature, poetry, and histology are also included. Volume 6 contains dissertations by his students, and the subsequent volumes (7–13) are mostly in Czech. English summaries of the contents are given in volumes 7–9. Purkinje's forgotten biological works, both published and unpublished, are the subject of volume 12. The final volume provides an overview of the contents of the previous ones and lists Purkinje's scientific works and discoveries. In addition, Kruta (the editor) presents a comprehensive biographical account of Purkinje's work. A full list (in English) of Purkinje's works, as well as responses to them, was also assembled by Kruta (1969).

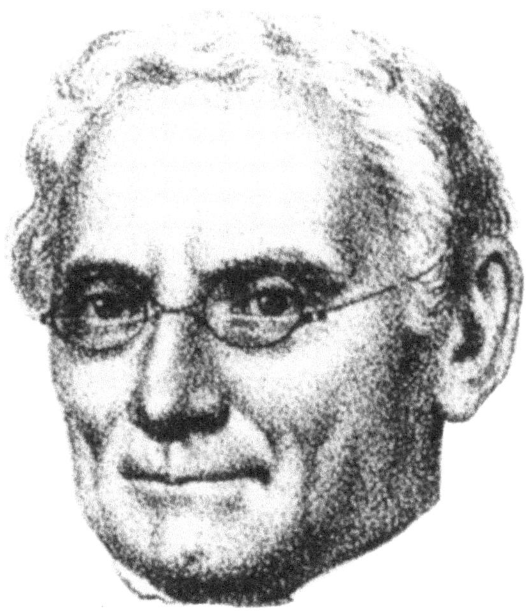

FIG. 2.4. Portrait of Purkinje, after an illustration kindly supplied by J. Hoskovec.

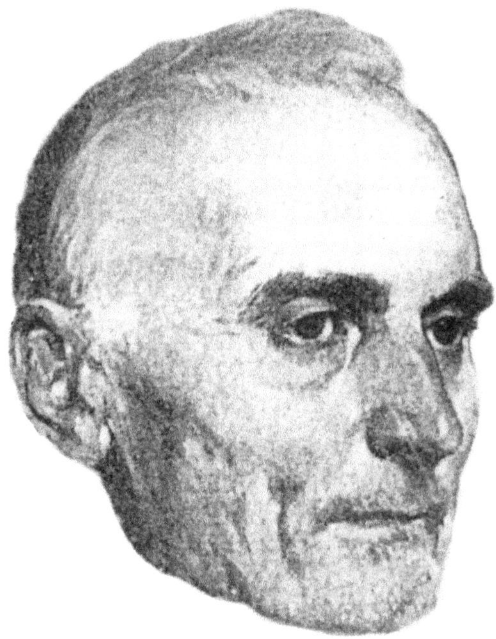

FIG. 3.1. Portrait of Purkinje in 1850, after an illustration in Purkinje's *Opera Omnia*, volume 6.

3

Historical Background for Research in Subjective Visual Phenomena

There are sensations which do not correspond to anything outside the body. In so far as they imitate the qualities and forms of external things, they thereby often give rise to illusions, phantoms, or appearances with no corresponding reality. These can be referred to as subjective sensory phenomena.

—Purkinje (1819/1823a, pp. 3–4)

INTRODUCTION

Subjective visual phenomena had a long history before Purkinje gave them that title, but he added greatly to the detail of their classification, description, and interpretation. The description of one's own sensations might seem the simplest of things to report on, but this is not the case. Helmholtz appreciated this only too well, and he commended Purkinje's special talent in this regard. Purkinje's doctoral dissertation, published in 1819, was entitled *Contributions to the Knowledge of Vision in its Subjective Aspect*. When it was reprinted in 1823 the title was extended to *Observations and Experiments on the Physiology of the Senses. Contributions to the Knowledge of Vision in its Subjective Aspect*. He commenced his research on visual phenomena because he had little access to equipment that would have allowed him to conduct experimental enquiries into other aspects of physiology. The second volume of *New Contributions*, which was dedicated to Goethe, appeared in 1825. As was noted in chapter 1, Goethe was both disappointed that Purkinje did not cite his own color research sufficiently and hopeful that Purkinje would advance phenomenological theory in an otherwise hostile climate among sensory physiologists. Their correspondence indicates the esteem in which Goethe was held by Purkinje, but also the independence of mind that the latter retained (see Kruta, 1966).

Despite the fact that many of the subjective phenomena examined by Purkinje had previously been described, his references to earlier observations were scant. His contribution was to classify the observations, describe them with precision, and interpret them within the context of the then known physiology. The first volume, which is translated in chapter 4 of this book, describes stroboscopic patterns, pressure figures, effects of galvanic stimulation, blind spot, pattern disappearances and distortions, visibility of retinal blood vessels and blood flow, afterimages, aftereffects, entoptic phenomena, single and double vision, and eye movements. The *New Contributions*, which were published in 1825, amplified several of the earlier topics but added some new ones, such as indirect vision, real and apparent motion, accommodation, near and far vision, and voluntary squinting. His preliminary estimations of color zones were included in the section on indirect vision, and what has become known as the Purkinje shift was described in a section concerned with color blending of afterimages and real images. The aim of this chapter is to provide an historical context into which Purkinje's (1819/1823a) observations can be placed. The topics are treated in approximately the order in which Purkinje described them, although the headings of the topics are generally briefer than those he applied. There is some overlap in the phenomena Purkinje described, and so some of them are conflated in the subsequent treatment. Such conflation can be determined from the roman numerals in parentheses applied to the topics, which correspond to those in chapter 4. Figure 3.2 shows the plate from Purkinje's book in which all the figures were presented.

LIGHT AND SHADE FIGURES (I)

The first phenomenon described by Purkinje was novel: He produced flicker, while looking at the bright sky, by waving his fingers in front of one eye and reported seeing checkerboards, zigzags, spirals, and ray patterns (see Fig. 3.2, Figs. 1–4). They were called shadow figures by Helmholtz (1867, 2000b) and are now referred to as stroboscopic patterns (Smythies, 1957), although they were described before the stroboscope was invented. When the eye is stimulated by an unpatterned, flickering light, patterns of bewildering complexity become visible. They are called

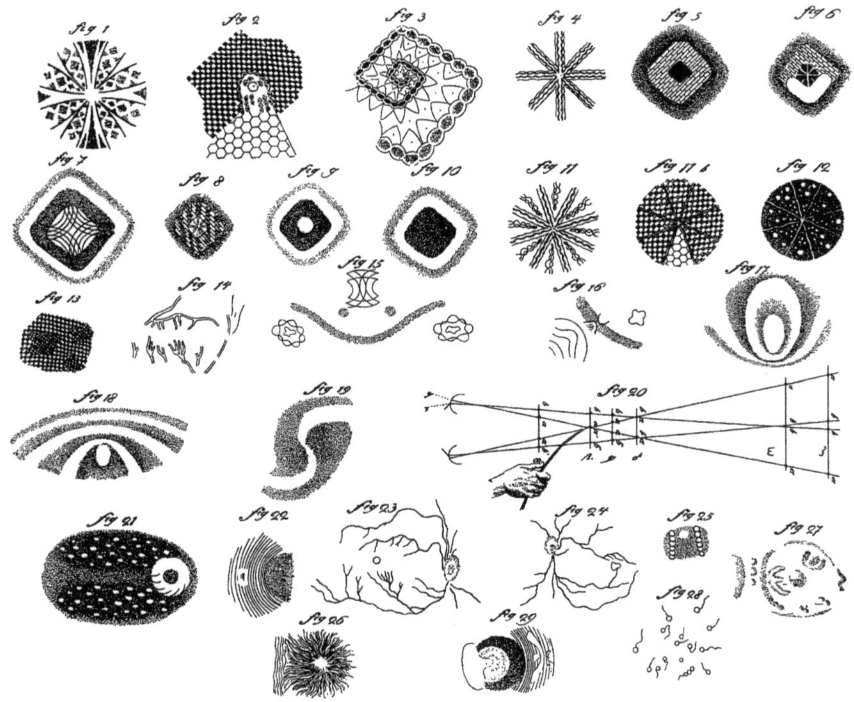

FIG. 3.2. The plate of figures appended to Purkinje (1819/1823a).

stroboscopic patterns after the modern form of the instrument, which can deliver pulses of light at very high frequencies.

The original stroboscopic disks, devised independently by Plateau and Stampfer in 1833, produced intermittent stimulation by means of a sequence of slits passing in front of the eye. Stroboscopic disks presented stimuli discretely, briefly, and in succession; that is, a sequence of drawings differing slightly from one another were viewed successively through slits in a rotating disk. To the astonishment of observers, a single figure appeared in motion: Perceived movement was synthesized from a sequence of still pictures. Stroboscopic disks were used to study visual persistence and apparent motion, and Purkinje made a variant of one in 1840; he called it the phorolyt, and it was sold commercially as a magic disk (Matousek, 1961).

Purkinje used his phorolyt to produce dynamic images of a range of natural movements generated from a sequence of static drawings. These ranged from the pumping action of the heart to the walking movements of newts; he also used it to display his own rotating posture (see Psotníčková, 1955). Two of these are shown in Fig. 3.3.

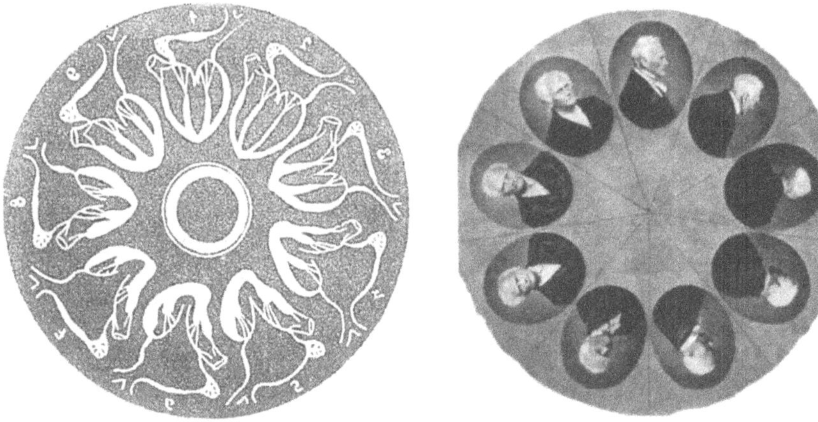

FIG. 3.3. Phorolyt pictures to show the action of the heart (left) and rotations of the head (right).

PRESSURE FIGURES (II, III, AND XXII)

The novelty of stroboscopic patterns contrasts with the antiquity of the next phenomena described by Purkinje—pressure figures. These figures were returned to several times in Purkinje's book, and so the other numbered sections describing the effects of pressure on the eye are indicated by the roman numerals in parentheses in the section headings. The pressure figures exhibited a wide range of manifestations (Fig. 3.2, Figs. 5–14). When pressure is applied to the eyeball, even in darkness, small patches of light are experienced; they have also been called phosphenes. They were described by Alcmaeon approximately 2,500 years ago (Stratton, 1917) and by many others in the intervening centuries. It is a very important phenomenon in the history of vision because it introduced the concept of emission of light from the eye, and subsequent writers sought to reconcile this aspect of seeing with the phenomena of optics (see Grüsser & Hagner, 1990; Park, 1997; Wade, 1998c); that is, the emission theories could be taken as having some empirical support, and no competing theory in antiquity could adequately account for the light seen in darkness as a consequence of a blow to the eye or pressure applied to it. The phenomenon has been reported many times, with occasional novelties of observation or interpretation.

A major refinement in the phenomenology of pressure figures was provided by Scheiner (1619). The phosphene was located opposite the point of pressure, and it could take on a variety of configurations; it could also be seen by day as well as in darkness, although the figures so generated were different. Scheiner believed that pressure generated some internal light that was reflected from the lens back to the retina. Descartes (1637/1902) provided a mechanistic interpretation of the phenomenon: The force on the optic nerve resulted in exciting the fibers in a similar way to light. For Newton (1717) the pressure figures were intensely colored, and they were transient, unless variations in the pressure exerted by the finger were introduced, an aspect confirmed by Elliott (1780) and Young (1793).

Descartes and Newton assigned the phenomenon to internal causes, but an empirical vindication of this was provided by Morgagni (1719). He generated pressure figures in his own eye in darkness and asked an assistant to note if any light could be seen issuing from his eye. In the absence of such light, Morgagni assumed that the figures were subjective and an index of healthy retinal function. He also extended the detail of description of the phenomenon: The characteristics of the phosphenes were dependent on the area and the pressure applied, and paired phosphenes could be produced. The checkered and streaky appearance of the pressure figures commented on by Purkinje was noted earlier by Elliott (1780), and Goethe (1810) drew attention to the light and dark circles that can be seen. Pressure figures were the first of only two visual phenomena mentioned by Elliott (1780), and his description was more vivid and elaborate than previous ones:

> After repeated trials, and putting myself to some pain, I learnt that by pressing the balls of my eyes with my hands, in the direction of their axes, with as much force as I could bear, keeping them steady, and assisting the pressure with the strong compression of the lids, and contraction of the neighbouring muscles, there would, after some time, appear a large luminous sensation like a concave hemisphere of light, but not very lucid, and chequered (often in a very regular manner) with dark and less lucid intervals. If the pressure be continued, and the eyes winked very strongly, the appearance will be much brighter, and will seem to tremble. There will sometimes also appear large crooked streaks of light, much brighter than the other parts, and with a certain vermicular, or eel-like motions. By increasing the pressure till the eyes become quite hot and red, the light will be brightest, and almost as lucid as at noon day: till this time the appearance is generally of a whitish colour, tinctured with yellow, or orange, like the sun; or rather like the light of the moon, or a candle. By continuing the extreme pressure, the brightness of the appearance begins to decay, and the colour gradually changes from a reddish and yellowish white, to a bluish one; and sometimes several kinds of coloured spots will appear, as red, green, blue, and a fine violet which generally disappears the last, and those more verging to red soonest; for now the light totally vanishes, nor can it be recalled by a continuation or increase of the pressure. If now the hands be removed, and the eyes opened, they will be quite blind even to the direct light of the sun; and it will be some time before they recover their sight, and then by degrees. (pp. 2–3)

Elliott even speculated on the basis for the checkered appearance: "The causes of which I take to be that the surface of the retina is not even or smooth, but has prominencies or ridges answerable to the regular form of the chequers, and which may result from its structure; so that the vitreous humour must press on it unequally, and by that means cause some parts of the appearance to look brighter, and others darker" (1780, p. 7).

None of these earlier reports was mentioned by Purkinje, who gave the most detailed account of the checkerboard figures, together with diagrams illustrating them.

GALVANIC LIGHT PHENOMENA (IV)

The effects of electrical stimulation on muscle contraction were discovered by Luigi Galvani in 1786 when he passed a discharge through isolated frog's legs (see Finger, 1994; Piccolino, 1997). This event is taken by some (e.g., Brazier, 1984, 1988) to mark the origin of neurophysiology. There followed numerous attempts to stimulate humans with electrical discharges, which were often applied to the whole head. In fact the procedure soon became a therapy for a wide range of medical conditions, and it was even administered to blind and deaf people. However, the theoretical significance of Galvani's experiments was his speculation that nerves transmitted electricity rather than animal spirit—the view that had been retained since antiquity. Galvani's experiments were confirmed by many and the term galvanic became synonymous with any electrical effects, whether produced by friction machines, by discharges from Leyden jars, or by currents from voltaic piles.

In the years following Galvani's discovery, most experimental attention was paid to the effects of electricity on excised muscle and nerve but some, like Alessandro Volta and Johann Ritter, applied currents to areas around the sense organs. One consequence that was soon appreciated from these experiments, as well as from therapeutic applications, was the visibility of light flashes following electrical stimulation in the region of the orbit. Volta (1800) reported that application of current (supplied by his newly invented battery) between the mouth and conjunctiva of the eye resulted in the experience of light, even in a dark room. Moreover, he noted that the visual sensation was associated with the onset and offset of the current, and a continuous impression of light could be produced by rapid alternation of polarity (see Piccolino, 2000). Ritter (1801, 1805) also reported that he could see colors filling the whole visual field with his eyes closed; if a zinc pole (cathode) was placed near the eye he saw blue light, and red was apparent with a copper pole (anode) so positioned. Moreover, objects could be discerned either more or less clearly with the eyes open, depending on the direction of the current. Neither Volta's nor Ritter's results were cited by Purkinje (1819/1823a), who conducted his experiments with a zinc pole in his mouth and a copper pole on his forehead. He reported patterns in addition to colors (see Fig. 3.2, Figs. 15 and 16), and these did not change with reversed polarity but they were dependent on the location of the electrodes.

INTRINSIC LIGHT AND GANZFELD EFFECTS (V AND VII)

The effects described by Purkinje under this heading are represented by Fig. 3.2, Figs. 17–19. They were referred to as the dark visual field and light chaos by Helmholtz (1867, 2000a) and they were also called the intrinsic light of the eye and *Eigengrau*—the experience of effects in the absence of all external light stimulation. Hering (1874) described it as mean gray, arguing that the experience of black occurs only with contrasting light stimulation. The conditions of unpatterned stimulation are essentially similar to those that constitute a Ganzfeld. Little attention had been paid to these phenomena before Purkinje's account. A distinguishing feature between the two effects is that scintillating points of light are more clearly visible with a Ganzfeld. The scintillations were similar to those observed with pressure and galvanic figures.

INTEROCULAR LIGHT EFFECTS (VI)

The cloudy streaks described by Purkinje under section V resulted from viewing with his right eye, as they were much more difficult to discern with his weaker left eye. It was estimated that Purkinje was myopic in his right eye and hyperopic and slightly astigmatic in his left eye; in his 30s, when these experiments would have been conducted, his right eye was said to require a 4-diopter correction (see Purkinje, 1958). In this section, he went on to describe the effects of differential light adaptation. When one eye was covered and the other exposed to a light surface for a minute, then afterwards the two visual fields struggled for dominance. This was a description of binocular rivalry, although Purkinje did not relate it to the previous work on this phenomenon.

Binocular rivalry occurs when the eyes are presented with radically different stimuli and it was described, albeit somewhat obliquely, by Porta (1593). The occurrence of alternating dominance was made more explicit by Le Clerc (1712) and Du Tour (1761), each of whom described the alternation between the rivaling targets. The former aligned two different objects binocularly by overconvergence, whereas the latter applied a prism to one eye. These are all instances of binocular contour rivalry; descriptions of color rivalry were given in the 18th century. Desaguliers (1716) facilitated overconvergence by viewing two differently colored patches of silk through an aperture. Du Tour (1760) achieved the same goal by fastening two differently colored fabrics on opposite sides of a septum placed between the eyes. Neither Desaguliers nor Du Tour mentioned longer visibility of one color or eye over the other, nor did Reid (1764), who combined the colors by means of two tubes.

Purkinje commenced the section by describing the consequences of passing from a bright into a dark place, but he made only passing comment to the process of dark adaptation itself. The momentary blindness to weak light after exposure to intense illumination seems so compelling that it must have been noticed from the earliest times, but there are relatively few reports of the phenomenon in the early literature. There are hints concerning its description in the works of Aristotle, Ibn al-Haytham, and Pecham (see Wade, 1998a), but they all have an element of ambiguity about them, unlike that of Francis Bacon (1627), which described both dark and light adaptation. Jurin (1738) judiciously excluded pupil dilation as the cause of dark adaptation on the basis of differences in time course; although the pupil adapts quickly to changes in illumination, the recovery from exposure to intense light requires much longer: "In coming out of a strong light, into a room with the window-shutters almost closed, we have an immediate sensation of darkness; and this continues much longer than the pupil requires to dilate and accomodate itself to that weak degree of light, which is almost instantly done. But after staying some time in a much darker place, the same room, which appeared dark before, will be sufficiently light" (pp. 169–170). Goethe (1810) suggested that there are differences in the duration of dark adaptation according to the strength of the eyes, and he did provide some values for the recovery period: "In passing from bright daylight to a dusky place we distinguish nothing at first: by degrees the eye recovers its susceptibility; strong eyes sooner than weak ones; the former in a minute, while the latter may require seven or eight minutes" (1840, p. 3).

BLIND SPOT (VIII, X, AND XI)

Purkinje devoted many pages to effects associated with the optic disk and blind spot in his first book on subjective vision. Unlike some of the other phenomena he described, there was no doubting its presence or the ease with which it could be demonstrated. It was both well known and well examined by the early 19th century. In addition to describing the effects for monocular and binocular viewing (VIII, Fig. 3.2, Fig. 20), Purkinje observed variations that are due to turning the eyes (X, Fig. 3.2, Figs. 21 and 22), and the light ring that is visible when a spot of light falls on the optic disk (XI).

The optic nerve and its insertion in the eye was clearly described by anatomists of antiquity, although its location was not accurately depicted before Scheiner (1619); prior to that the optic nerve was shown as leaving the eye on the optic axis. At approximately the same time Kepler (1604, 1611) demonstrated how an image is formed on the retina, and Platter (1583) earlier argued for the retina as the receptive organ, but physiologists in the late 17th century raised doubts about this conclusion. The doubts were based on a compelling phenomenon, first described by Mariotte (1668), namely the blind spot. Mariotte found that the image of a small object falling on the base of the optic nerve is invisible when one eye alone is used. The phenomenon enabled Mariotte and others to locate the optic nerve with precision, either in terms of visual angles or retinal dimensions. Harris (1775) measured the angular separation of the blind spot from the optic axis in two people and gave a value of 14°–15°. Young (1801), with his precise and mathematical approach, gave the diameter of the optic disk as 1/30 of an inch and its distance from the visual axis as 16/100 of an inch.

Smith (1738) carried out experiments on the visibility of the blind spot and implicated binocular processes in its normal invisibility. "So far Mr. *Mariotte*; whose experiment I have tryed in a chamber from which all sensible light was excluded, except what came into it through a key-hole; and this also disappeared totally when it fell upon the base of the optick nerve; which shews it to be totally insensitive to light. Yet in looking at objects of an uniform colour with one eye, we are not sensible of any such defect or dark round spot... This defect of sensation having been constantly supplyed by the other eye, is now supplyed by the imagination only" (Smith, 1738, *Remarks*, p. 7). Purkinje did make reference to this last observation in a translation of Smith's book into German (Smith, 1755).

Purkinje argued that the optic disk is not without some small degree of sensitivity. The evidence for this was derived from the observation that, although a small light falling on the optic disk disappears, it produces a halo around the optic disk, which appears to move in the opposite direction to that of the light.

PATTERN DISAPPEARANCES WITH STEADY FIXATION OUTSIDE THE BLIND SPOT (IX)

Purkinje extended the observations on the blind spot by examining pattern disappearances outside the blind spot. The disappearance of peripheral patterns when one is maintaining fixation on a central one is often referred to as the Troxler effect, after Troxler's (1804) description to which Purkinje referred. Troxler arranged a sequence of color patches on a wall so that they extended into the periphery of vision. When he fixated on one, after some time the most peripheral ones disappeared, followed by those closer to the fixation point. In all cases, the lost patterns were replaced with the blue wall, which was the background. A decade before Troxler, Erasmus Darwin (1794) observed a similar fading and then disappearance of centrally fixated targets. He made this discovery in the context of his experiments on afterimages, which demanded prolonged fixation of color patches in order for them to be rendered visible. During the prolonged fixation the intensity of the color declined until the whole patch ceased to be visible. Brewster (1818), on the other hand, maintained that fixated objects never disappeared, whereas peripheral ones did, even when viewed binocularly. For Purkinje the patterns were replaced with cloudy streaks, rather like some of the effects seen with stroboscopic patterns. How he was able to conduct the experiment described is a puzzle, as the act of blowing the pieces of paper away would have resulted in some eye or head movement, and such movements are known to restore faded images. He elaborated the conditions and descriptions associated with pattern disappearances.

LIGHT HALOS (XII)

When a bright light, like a candle flame, is viewed against a dark background, halos and radiations become visible. Purkinje's description of these effects might have been in part a consequence of astigmatism. A similar description and similar illustrations were provided by Young (1801), who measured astigmatism in his own eye. A small spot of light was not seen as such, and it varied in shape according to the distance that it was from the eye:

> When I look at a minute lucid point, such as the image of a candle in a small concave speculum, it appears as a radiated star, as a cross, or as an unequal line, and never as a perfect point, unless I apply a concave lens inclined at a proper angle, to correct the unequal refraction of my eye. If I bring the point very near, it spreads into a surface nearly circular, and almost equably illuminated, except some faint lines, nearly in a radiating direction. (pp. 43–44).

Purkinje made reference to Young's article in his *New Contributions*, but it was not mentioned in the context of the light halos. Turbidity of the media in the eye was one of the interpretations Purkinje suggested, although this was thought to be a characteristic of the retina as well as the ocular media.

RETINAL BLOOD VESSELS (THE PURKINJE TREE) (XIII)

Interest in the visibility of retinal blood vessels arose from conflicts concerning the blind spot. Mariotte (1668) concluded that the choroid rather than the retina was the surface receptive to light. Pecquet (1668) disputed this conclusion, but was surprised that a phenomenon as compelling as the blind spot had not previously been recorded. The dispute introduced another novel and compelling phenomenon, the previous ignorance of which is similarly remarkable. Pecquet argued that the blood vessels of the retina prevent light's passing to both the retina and the choroid and therefore they should be visible. Moreover, because the blood vessels were larger at their trunk (the optic disk) than in the axis of vision they were not considered to pose a problem for central vision. La Hire (1694) presented a diagram that could be taken to represent the large vessels near the optic disk (see chapter 5), although his description of the phenomenon was in the context of seeing floaters in the eye.

Bell (1803) realized that the visible ramifications were shadows on the retina cast by the vessels: "There is a kind of umbræ seen before the eyes which are occasioned by the vessels of the retina . . . the person sees umbrageous ramifications which strike across the sphere of vision, and are synchronous with the pulse, showing its dependance on the full and throbbing pulsation of the head" (p. 295). Purkinje specified their characteristics in greater detail and illustrated their appearance (Fig. 3.2, Figs. 23 and 24). Indeed, the pattern is often called the Purkinje tree, after Purkinje's description and illustration of the ramifications. Wheatstone (C.W., 1830), in his review of Purkinje's book, devised an even better method for rendering the vessels visible. Directing a narrow, moving beam of light into the corner of the eye, he noted that the shadows moved in the direction opposite to the light source; if the motion stopped, the ramifications fragmented and disappeared. Of greater significance was the crescent-shaped shadow cast by the fovea. He demonstrated that this region did correspond to the center of the visual axis by generating a foveal afterimage and then locating it with respect to the crescent shadow. Thus Wheatstone was using an afterimage as a stabilized retinal image in order to define the relative location of other retinal structures. He suggested a slightly different procedure for observing the finer vessels: A card with a large pinhole was moved by the side of the eye so that diffuse light could enter the eye. Wheatstone could not see any vessels around the fovea, and he referred to the "differences of colour observed by anatomists," which was an allusion to Soemmerring's (1801) yellow spot.

AFTERIMAGES AND VISUAL PERSISTENCE (XIV)

Afterimages can be seen following either brief, intense illumination of the eye or prolonged fixation on an illuminated stimulus. Thus, looking briefly at a bright light, like a candle flame, can result in its continued visibility when the eyes are closed or directed away from the light to a uniform surface. They have been referred to as ocular spectra and accidental colors, both of which refer to the colored characteristics of the phenomenon. Purkinje called them *Blendungsbilder*, which term was used to include not only afterimages from intense illumination but also persisting images of moving lights. They were probably combined under one heading because Purkinje examined the interaction between the afterimages and the surfaces onto which they were projected; they did indeed blend with the background.

The term afterimage (*Nachbild*) itself was used by Purkinje in the final section (XXVIII) of his book, and it was taken up by Fechner (1840) in his more detailed study of them, although the two visual scientists did not apply it in the same way. There are numerous accounts of afterimages before Purkinje, and they have posed constant problems for accounts of vision (see Wade, 1978a). Franz (1899) summarized the situation succinctly: "In the history of after-images we seem to have an epitome of the interrelations of physics, physiology and psychology; and probably no other single phenomenon is so good an example of the growth of experiment and measurement in psychology" (p. 1).

One stimulus used by Purkinje was a candle flame that could be viewed briefly or for prolonged periods; after looking at it and covering his eyes, he saw first a positive, then a negative, afterimage. The effects of brief, intense stimulation were considered first, and Purkinje described the sequence of afterimages that followed. This sequence was the source of intense interest in the late 19th and early 20th centuries, and the second positive phase of the afterimage became known as the Purkinje afterimage (see Judd, 1927). The afterimages following brief observation of very intense light sources, like the Sun, resulted in much longer positive phases. Those generated by prolonged fixation of a candle flame passed through a similar sequence of colors, but more gradually.

Another technique Purkinje adopted was to form a patterned afterimage by fixation on a paned window. The procedure had been described by Aguilonius (1613), who noted that subsequently viewing a uniform surface, like white paper, yielded a negative afterimage; that is, the parts of the afterimage that corresponded to the glass panes looked dark, whereas the bars appeared brighter. In the 17th century Castelli pursued this in a more systematic manner in a remarkable study of afterimages that also set out a number of their critical features (see Ariotti, 1973). He used a stimulus (a lead-framed window) that afforded good fixation: When the eyes were closed, the afterimage retained the shape of the window and it passed through a sequence of colors. The visibility of the afterimage was itself cyclical: It faded from view, only to reappear and fade again. When the eyes were open, the apparent size of the afterimage varied with the distance of the surface onto which it was projected. This last observation was made with greater precision in the late 19th century (Emmert, 1881), and it is commonly referred to as Emmert's law. Castelli commented on this aspect of the apparent size of afterimages, as did Robert Darwin (1786).

Many of the early reports of afterimages followed fixation on naturally occurring bright objects, like the Sun, although this was likely to damage the eye. Purkinje was not averse to subjecting his body to abnormal stimulation for the sake of science, and he adopted this technique too. He had illustrious predecessors: Newton (1691/1829) viewed the Sun's image reflected in a mirror "with the hazard of my eyes." He might well have damaged his eyesight since the "phantasm" he reported remained visible long after the initial observation of the Sun. Newton noted that the visibility of the afterimage could be extended by winking and that it seemed to be influenced by attention. What is of particular significance is that he conducted the first experiment on interocular transfer: he could see the afterimage when using his left eye, even though it had been induced in the right eye. The transferred afterimage was said to be "almost as plain" as the monocular one. Newton did see colors, but his report did not dwell on them or their sequence.

General characteristics of afterimages were elucidated by both Jurin (1738) and Buffon (1743). Jurin proposed the principle of reciprocal action on the basis of the variations visible in long-lasting afterimages. For example, the afterimage of a window was in opposite contrast to that seen under normal viewing, and so the processes in the retina that produced the afterimage were the reverse of those generated by the primary stimulus. Buffon stated a similar relation with respect to colored afterimages: Objects of one color (say red) produce afterimages that are complementary (green). Buffon introduced the term accidental colors to distinguish them from the perception of natural colors. An interpretation of such accidental colors was advanced by Scherffer (1761). Any colored stimulus will produce a strong effect for that color and a weaker one at other colors; following intense stimulation, there is a loss of sensibility, and viewing a white surface will result in a more powerful influence of the previously more weakly stimulated color. The afterimages were said to be more intense when the natural color was viewed against a black background and then projected onto a white surface. In addition, Scherffer indicated that accidental colors mixed in a way similar to that of natural colors: He placed a red and a yellow square next to one another and alternately fixated them; when a white surface was subsequently viewed, three afterimages were evident—a greenish-blue in the center, flanked by green and violet squares.

Franklin (1765/1970) provided a quantitative note by indicating the duration for which afterimages remained visible: Colors faded faster than shapes, which could last for many seconds. Purkinje examined the relationship between the duration of an afterimage and the prior fixation. The general principle obtained was that the afterimage of a candle lasted for 20 times the period of prior observation. He also found that the negative afterimage of the candle was visible long after the colors had faded from view.

A clear distinction between positive and negative afterimages was made by Robert Darwin (1786). He made a series of observations on this and other phenomena. He used a simple black "tadpole" shape on white paper to generate the afterimage. A negative afterimage could be seen on the white paper, and it appeared whiter than the paper itself. His interpretation of this effect was, essentially, in terms of differential retinal adaptation. The visibility of afterimages could be revived by intermittent stimulation (moving the hand in front of the eyes), and it was noted that there can be a latency before the afterimage is initially visible (see Wade, 1978a).

Purkinje added an element of quantification to studies of afterimages by determining a relationship between the duration of visibility of the afterimage and of the initial period of observation. He also described the sequence of colors that are briefly visible after intense stimulation. In addition, Purkinje included, under the heading *Blendungsbilder*, those less intense images that persist for longer than the physical presence of the stimulus, like a rotating top or ember. This is a phenomenon of great antiquity, but Purkinje restricted most of his discussion to Newton's rotating color disk.

Under normal circumstances the moving luminous objects we observe can be resolved during their motion, either because they move slowly or because they can be pursued by the eyes. Certain naturally occuring events (like comets and lightning) do not satisfy these conditions, and they were commented on in antiquity (see Wade, 1998a). Aristotle discussed persisting images in general, and he likened the effects to those of a projectile moving through space. Seneca (63/1971) gave an account of shooting stars that is remarkable because it attributed the visible trail to the "slowness of vision" rather than to any attribute of the object itself. Ptolemy used the same principle implicitly in devising a color top, and he made explicit reference to the visibility of rapidly rotating disks and wheels. He also mentioned briefly a simple method of demonstrating persisting images (and the one chosen by Purkinje), namely a rapidly moving flame: "Examples are to be found in a fire that moves for a brief time, a spark, and [luminous] bodies that pass by windows and narrow openings" (Smith, 1996, p. 123).

Ibn al-Haytham rotated Ptolemy's flame to generate a theme that was replayed constantly throughout the following centuries: Rapid motion of a burning stick results in the visibility of the path through which it passes. Leonardo drew circles of flame in this way; he also added the subtle variation of moving the eyes with respect to a fixed flame, with a similar visual effect (see MacCurdy, 1938). Newton (1717) appreciated that the phenomenon could be employed to measure the duration of the persisting images. He suggested that its value was less than a second, but precise measurements were made by Chevalier D'Arcy (1765): "For this purpose he contrived a machine, which consisted of a cross, turning horizontally upon its center, by means of a wheel and a weight, the velocity of which he could vary at pleasure, and ascertain to the utmost exactness. To view this machine, he placed an observer at 28 toises [approximately 55 m] from it, in a room in which no light was admitted but what came from the object (which was a live coal fastened upon the cross) and the experiments were made in the night time.... He found that the coal seemed to make an uninterrupted circle, when it revolved in 8 thirds of a minute [8/60 s]; and that no velocity less than this would answer the purpose. It made no difference at whatever distance from the center of the cross the coal was placed, or whether the machine was viewed through a telescope, or in any other manner he could think of applying. The result was also the same, at whatever distance the machine was viewed" (Priestley, 1772, pp. 634–635). D'Arcy's estimate of visual persistence was approximately 130 ms—a value that corresponds closely to those subsequently obtained with more modern devices.

Robert Darwin (1786) elaborated on an aspect of visual persistence described by Leonardo: Brief exposure of parts of a single figure (if the intervals between them are sufficiently short) results in the visibility of the whole figure. Darwin's observations were more acute because he noted that the brightness of the scene seen through a rotating sail was less than that without the sail. Wheatstone (1827) made a more elaborate device with rotating sectors for viewing pictures, the parts of which were successively exposed. Wheatstone's concerns with visual persistence were stimulated by his research in acoustics, and particularly by Young's (1800) description of vibrating piano strings: "Take one of the lowest strings of a square piano forte, round which a fine silvered wire is wound in a spiral form; contract the light of a window, so that, when the eye is placed in the proper position, the image of the light may appear small, bright, and well defined, on each of the convolutions of the wire. Let the chord be now made to vibrate, and the luminous point will delineate its path like a burning coal whirled round, and will present to the eye a line of light, which, by the assistance of a microscope, may be accurately observed" (p. 135).

PATTERN DISTORTIONS (XV–XVII)

The three phenomena described by Purkinje under the heading pattern distortions are seen with high-contrast regular geometrical patterns, like parallel lines or concentric circles. Erasmus Darwin (1796) described the dizziness that can result from looking at patterned wallpaper and how this can be suppressed: “In a room hung with paper, which is coloured over with similar small black lozenges or rhomboids, many people become dizzy; for when they begin to fall, the next and the next lozenge succeeds upon the eye; which they mistake for the first, and are not aware, that they have any apparent motion. But if you fix a sheet of paper, or draw any other figure, in the midst of these lozenges, the charm ceases, and no dizziness is perceptible—The same occurs, when we ride over a plain covered with snow without trees or other eminent objects” (p. 233).

Copper engravings produced patterns with very fine lines in them, and they were used by Purkinje to examine some distortions that accompany prolonged fixation. Moving the patterns produced blurred streaks, the orientation of which was dependent on the direction of motion. These scintillating clouds were also evident during steady fixation on the lines, and they could obliterate visibility of the physical stimulus (XV). After some seconds of such observation, shimmering patterns were visible when the eyes were closed (XVI). He also noted that patterns of finely engraved parallel lines lose their straightness with prolonged viewing (XVII). His descriptions initiated a wide range of other studies that continue to the present. The distortions have not only proved to be of interest to visual scientists but visual artists have also manipulated them (see Wade 1977b, 1982, 1990, 1998d; Wilkins, 1995). The distorting effects are not restricted to parallel lines but can be seen more vividly in patterns of concentric circles, as Purkinje noted. When the circles are moved back and forth, shadowy segments are visible, and these can be related to the direction of motion.

Stationary concentric circles provide a different type of distortion to parallel lines: Cloudy streaks appear to radiate from the center, and they can themselves rotate. Purkinje associated these effects with variations in accommodation, although he did not say how they were related. The distortions were radial with concentric circles and circular with a pattern of radiating lines (see Fig. 3.4), that is, they were perpendicular to the lines in the pattern. In the *New Contributions* Purkinje wrote the following (1825a):

> One draws a series of closely spaced concentric circles, constructed as neatly as possible.... These are displaced outside the distance of distinct vision, and there appear in all directions bands of clearly distinguishable parallel lines, over which the multitude of lines slide and entwine as cloudy streaks and points; they all radiate from the center to the periphery, and their number, width and direction differ with different individuals, but remain constant for any one.... One can produce the same appearance very clearly with a figure comprised of 16 or more radii. (pp. 144–145)

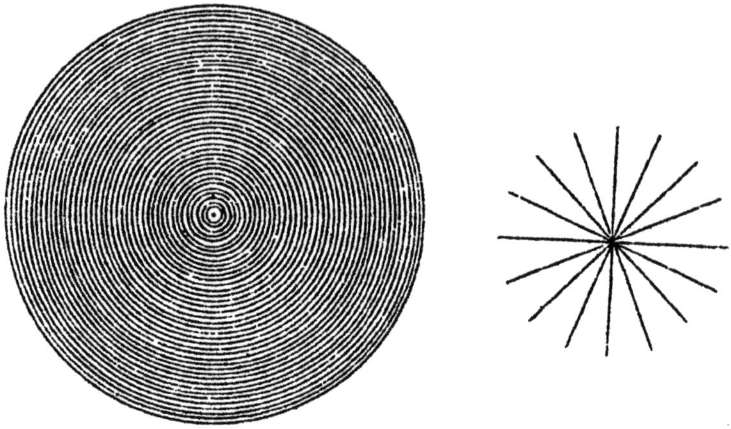

FIG. 3.4. Concentric circles and ray figures as illustrated in Purkinje (1825a).

Such effects can be attributed to transient forms of astigmatism that are a consequence of instabilities in the ciliary muscles (Wade, 1977b).

It is not clear from Purkinje's descriptions whether observation was monocular or binocular; in his case it might not have made too much difference because he had a marked difference in the acuity of his eyes, with the right being much stronger than the left. He attributed the apparent waviness of the straight lines to the overlap of the real image of the lines with a displaced afterimage, after the manner of moiré or interference fringes.

The distortions described under sections XV and XVII occur during observation of the regular geometrical patterns whereas those under XVI are successive. The zigzag motion over a blank field is rather like a motion aftereffect but there is no physical motion that precedes it. The zigzag motion described by Purkinje was seen following fixation on a stationary pattern. If it consisted of fine, regular, parallel lines, then prolonged observation produced an aftereffect of motion perpendicular to the lines in the adapting pattern. This aftereffect has been rediscovered many times since, and it is now called the complementary aftereffect (see Wade, 1977b, 1982). The shimmering movement is also visible during stimulation, particularly with radiating patterns with blank annuli in them. Such stimuli have been used in brain imaging studies to determine the cortical location that is most active during the perceived motion (Zeki, Watson, & Frackowiak, 1993).

VOLUNTARY MOVEMENT OF THE PUPIL (XVIII)

Variations in pupil size with accommodation have been noted since Scheiner (1619), but little attention had been paid to its voluntary control until Whytt (1763) devoted a chapter of his book to variations in pupil size. Purkinje trained himself to focus on two points at different distances with the corresponding changes in pupil diameter—smaller for near and larger for far. He then performed the same task without the points' being present, with the same results.

ENTOPTIC PHENOMENA (XIX–XXI AND XXIII)

Entoptic phenomena are taken to refer to the visible expression of structures within the eye itself, and Purkinje made several observations on them. Visibility of the retinal blood vessels (XIII) could be included here but they have had a more specific observational history, and they were treated separately by Purkinje. The phenomena under this heading have basked in an array of graphic appellations. They stem mostly from the Latin *muscae volitantes*, which term could have derived from the description given by Grassus in the 12th century (see Wood, 1929). They have been translated into *mouches volantes*, *fliegende Mücken*, *flying gnats*, or, much more prosaically, *floaters*. All refer to seeing inclusions in the eye, which are most clearly visible against a bright, unpatterned background. Because they are usually in peripheral vision and in relatively fixed locations, any attempts to fixate on them results in their corresponding motion, hence the name. Purkinje reported seeing several at the same time and described their motion as that of falling stars (XXI).

Early in the 17th century, Platter observed a spot before his eye one day and gave a precise interpretation of its cause: Debris from the ciliary processes floated freely in the aqueous humor, blocking the light entering the eye (see Koelbing, 1967). Willis (1664) remarked on the phenomenon, which he had frequently encountered in his medical examinations, and assigned its cause to blockages in the fibers of the optic nerve. La Hire (1694) distinguished between two types of *mouches volantes*: One retained a fixed visual direction, and the other appeared to move about; they were more readily seen by presbyopes. As noted above, La Hire's illustration bore a closer resemblance to the retinal blood vessels around the optic disk than to Purkinje's drawing of *mouches volantes*.

Boerhaave (1703) and Robert Darwin (1786) commented on a much more subtle entoptic feature—the circulation of the blood in the retinal blood vessels. According to Darwin: "By being accustomed to observe such small sensations in the eye, it is easy to see the circulation of the blood in this organ. I have attended to this frequently, when I have observed my eyes more than commonly sensible to other spectra. The circulation may be seen either in both eyes at a time, or only in one of them" (p. 344). Purkinje also described and illustrated the circulation of blood in the eye (XX, Fig. 3.2, Fig. 25). After vigorous exercise, a variety of shapes can be seen when looking at a large unpatterned surface, like the clear sky. The circles that are seen seem to pulsate in synchrony with the pulse itself, and they can be rendered clearer when pressure is applied to the eye (XXIII).

Helmholtz (1867, 2000b) devoted a chapter to entoptic phenomena, but Purkinje's observations were mentioned only in the context of the retinal blood vessels, and then only in the historical section.

FIREY RINGS (XXIV)

The earlier work of Eichel (1774) and a translation of Elliott's (1780) *Philosophical Observations on the Senses of Vision and Hearing* (Elliott, 1785) are cited in connection with the seven phenomena listed under this heading. They tend to be related to the pressure figures and effects surrounding the optic disk. As mentioned in the third section of this chapter, Elliott described pressure figures in some detail, but we have not been able to consult Eichel's work to read about his observations of the firey rings.

SINGLE AND DOUBLE VISION (XXV)

Many of the phenomena described by Purkinje were observed with his right eye because of the marked difference between the acuity of his eyes. He wrote relatively little about binocular vision but he did include a section on single and double vision. These topics have been perhaps of more constant interest to students of vision than any other (see Howard & Rogers, 1995). Despite this continuity of concern over many centuries, the use of two eyes to derive stereoscopic depth perception was not appreciated until after Purkinje had completed his own observations and experiments. In the 1830s Wheatstone invented an instrument, the stereoscope, that radically altered both our picture of vision and our vision of pictures. Prior to his contributions to the physiology of vision, the sole concern of investigations in binocular vision was singleness rather than depth (see Wade, 1987). Purkinje followed in this path, and it is of interest to note that Purkinje's section on binocular vision was not included in the summary of his book written by Wheatstone (C.W., 1830).

Observations on the differences between vision with one eye and two have been recorded since antiquity (see Wade, 1998b), but experimental enquiries into binocular vision were initiated by Ptolemy (ca. 150). He appreciated that monocular and binocular visual directions were not necessarily the same. To confirm this empirically, he constructed a board on which he could place vertical rods at different distances in the midline (see Howard & Wade, 1996). He provided a description of one of the most commonly used examples of crossed and uncrossed visual directions: With fixation on the far rod, the nearer one appeared double, and to the left with the right eye and to the right with the left eye; the reverse occurred with fixation on the nearer rod. Ptolemy stated that singleness of vision with two eyes occurred when the two visual directions corresponded, thus introducing the concept of correspondence into binocular vision. He modified his board to take three rods and found that objects appeared single to two eyes when they were in the same plane as the fixation point. These facts were interpreted in terms of the visual axes and the common axis. Ibn al-Haytham made a similar board on which he placed wax cylinders, but of different colors (see Sabra, 1989).

In the second century Galen introduced the method of separating the two eyes by means of a septum and reported that vision of a peripheral target seen by one eye when both were open was inferior to that with one eye alone (see May, 1968). This position was to be repeatedly maintained until the 17th century, and it accorded with Galenic theory that the visual spirit, the source of which was at the optic chiasm, was more concentrated when one eye was open than when both were in use. In similarly placing the visual faculty at the chiasm, Roger Bacon made the analogy of singleness of vision to a fountain: Because a fountain has but one source, so is vision with two eyes single (Burke, 1928). Galen's method of separating the two eyes was applied with good effect by Porta (1593) in the context of eye dominance, and Porta also illustrated Galen's description of the apparent locations of an object seen with each eye separately and with both eyes. Porta stepped out of the Galenic mold by proposing a theory of single vision that was both parsimonious and supported by the phenomenon of binocular rivalry: We see singly with two eyes by using only one at once. Porta's suppression theory could be contrasted with fusion theories of the type advanced by Aguilonius (1613), who introduced the term *horopter*.

Descartes' (1637/1902, 1664/1909) analysis of binocular vision was by analogy to a blind man's locating an object with two sticks, and Newton (1682, see Turnbull, 1960) emphasized the notion of retinal correspondence in determining binocular single vision. Smith (1738) both described and illustrated crossed and uncrossed retinal disparities, but their role in stereoscopic vision was overlooked. Smith's book was translated into German and it was cited in other contexts by Purkinje, but not regarding binocular vision. Wells (1792) conducted experimental investigations into the characteristics of binocular visual direction by using apertures and also different colored threads extending from each eye to a common point. Ptolemy had constructed a similar arrangement with one of his boards on which colored lines were drawn from the eyes to pass through a common point of intersection. Wells' (1792) *Essay on single vision with two eyes* was one of the first books dedicated to binocular vision, and it is replete with excellent experiments, although stereoscopic vision was not mentioned.

STARING VAGUELY INTO THE DISTANCE (XXVI)

Very little is added under this heading other than the description of the effects that accompany the relaxed state of the eyes.

EYE MOVEMENTS (XXVII)

One of the most readily observable aspects of vision is the way the eyes move, and this is a topic that has a long descriptive history. Purkinje commenced with the long known relationship between eye movements and distinct vision, but he did discuss the difference in the ease with which the eyes could move in different directions. There was reference to the short and rapid movements that occur with relaxed eyes in darkness, and he related these to eye movements in blind people. Purkinje did note the differences in ocular demeanor associated with insane and feeble-minded people. Indeed, he regarded the characteristics of eye movements as reflecting the essence of humanity.

The involuntary movements that attend fixation were reported by Mariotte (1683), and Robert Darwin (1786) provided an expression of this in the formation of afterimages. The function that eye movements served was also stressed by many writers—namely to direct the eyes to objects of interest, so that they can be seen distinctly. The rapid inspection of objects by a succession of eye movements was detailed by Scheiner (1619), Porterfield (1737, 1759), Harris (1775), and Young (1801), who gave the range over which the eye could move. Porterfield treated eye movements in a manner very similar to that adopted later by Purkinje. His experiments and analysis of accommodation were described in chapter 1. Porterfield appreciated that as acuity declined with retinal eccentricity then it would be difficult to perceive clearly all parts of a large object at once. Accordingly, he considered that vision was dependent on a person's scanning objects by moving the eyes. A second factor that was implicated in this was the importance of visual persistence in yielding a unified percept during scanning (1737):

> Now, though it is certain that only a very small Part of any Object can at once be clearly and distinctly seen, namely, that whose Image on the *Retina* is in the *Axis* of the Eye; and that the other Parts of the Object, which have their Images painted at some Distance from this same *Axis*, are but faintly and obscurely perceived, and yet we are seldom sensible of this Defect; and, in viewing any large Body, we are ready to imagine that we see at the same Time all its Parts equally distinct and clear: But this is a vulgar Error, and we are led into it from the quick and almost continual Motion of the Eye, whereby it is successively directed towards all the Parts of the Object in an Instant of Time. (pp. 185–186)

Porterfield's two essays on motions of the eyes were expanded in his *Treatise*, published two decades later; Purkinje (1825a) did cite Porterfield's *Treatise* when addressing vertigo (see chapter 1), but Porterfield was not referred to in the context of the study of eye movements.

The movements of the eyes that are both easier to observe in others and to produce oneself are voluntary. Both eyes generally move together, and this was a feature commented on by Aristotle (Ross, 1927). The eyes are, of course, moved by muscles, and Galen gave a lucid account of the six extraocular muscles, describing the three axes around which the eye can rotate (see May, 1968). Descartes (1662) provided a speculative mechanistic account of how the paired muscles work by means of reciprocal action.

More methodological studies were initiated by Wells (1792), who used an afterimage as a stabilized retinal image. Not only did he examine the characteristics of postrotary nystagmus (see chapter 1), but he implicated eye movements in visual direction. The direction in which an object appears is not determined by visual stimulation alone, as it also involves information about the position of the eyes—otherwise objects would appear to move with every movement of the eyes. Helmholtz (1867, 2000c) made a distinction between what have become called outflow and inflow theories. The former refers to deriving eye movement information from efferent (centrally generated) impulses to the eye muscles, whereas the latter reflects use of afferent (sensory) signals from the eye muscles themselves. How this compensation for eye rotation comes about has been a matter of considerable enquiry, the origins of which can be found in the late 18th century. Robert Darwin and Wells feature again in this arena, but not disputatiously.

One way of examining the association between eye and image movements is to sever the link between them. This can be done by means of a stabilized retinal image, and the afterimage provided the earliest approach to this. Robert Darwin's (1786) observation was fortuitous: having formed a peripheral afterimage, he sought to examine it, but each eye movement in pursuit of it resulted in its apparent motion in the direction of the eye movement. If the eye remained stationary, then so did the afterimage. No theoretical implications were made regarding this by Darwin, unlike Wells (1792), who appreciated fully the import of this and similar observations that he made himself. He conducted the following experiment (1792):

> Having looked steadily for some time at the flame of a candle, with *one* eye only, I directed afterward, with both eyes open, my attention to the middle of a sheet of paper, a few feet distant; the consequence of which was, that a spot appeared upon it in the same manner, as if I had viewed the flame with both eyes, though somewhat fainter. My attention remaining fixed upon the sheet, I now pushed the eye, by which the spot was seen, successively upward and downward, to the right and to the left, and in every oblique direction; The spot however never altered its position, but kept constantly upon the middle of the appearance of the paper, perceived by the undistorted eye, though the appearance of the paper to the distorted eye, was always separate from the former, and the sheet consequently seen double. . . . The apparent situation of the spot being . . . at the same time affected by the *voluntary* motions of the eye, it must, I think, be necessarily owing to the *action* of the muscles by which these motions are performed. (pp. 68–70)

In short, Wells provided experimental support for outflow theory (see Ono, 1981). Bell (1823) confirmed the distinction between the effects of voluntary and involuntary eye movements on afterimage motion (see Wade, 1978a, 1978b).

IMAGINATION AND MEMORY IMAGES (XXVIII)

Afterimages, which Purkinje also referred to as *Blendungsbilder*, have properties different from those of the *Nachbild* described in the final section. The section starts with a further reference to persisting images, namely those that render vision continuous during blinking. This aspect of visual persistence was commented on by Locke (1690): "How frequently do we, in a day, cover our Eyes with our Eyelids, without perceiving that we are at all in the dark?" (p. 63). He related this to the continued visibility of rotating objects and provided an interpretation in terms of his associationist theory of mind. The absence of any visible effects of blinking was given a more physiological account by Erasmus Darwin (1794): "So we many times in an hour cover our eye-balls with our eye-lids without perceiving that we are in the dark; hence the perception or idea of light is not changed for that of darkness in so small a time as the twinkling of an eye; so that in this case the muscular motion of the eye-lid is performed quicker than the perception of light can be changed for that of darkness" (p. 24). Because Darwin's book had been translated into German and was cited in the case of vertigo, it is surprising that no mention of him is made with regard to this phenomenon.

Both afterimages and memory images appear to be projected outside the eye, but Purkinje distinguished between them on the basis of their relationships to eye movements: Afterimages move with the eye, whereas memory images remain stable in space. This is another instance in which a knowledge of the older literature would have been an advantage to Purkinje. The ways in which afterimages appear to move depend on the nature of the eye movements—they move with voluntary eye movements but not with passive ones. This was established by Wells (1792) in a series of subtle experiments.

It is in the context of memory images that Purkinje makes one of his rare forays into the brain itself. Ideas about cortical localization were widely debated in the early 19th century (see Wade, 2000d). Gall and Spurzheim (1810) combined their anatomical knowledge with psychological speculation in proposing a system of organology (which others later called phrenology), localizing cognitive functions in specific cortical areas. Purkinje was very cautious about these views as he did not consider that enough was known about the brain to justify such theorizing. It is strange that one who was to add so much to knowledge of neural function at the microscopic level was so reticent to speculate about brain activity at the macroscopic level. Purkinje concludes with displaying his romantic physiology by relating all the senses to the soul.

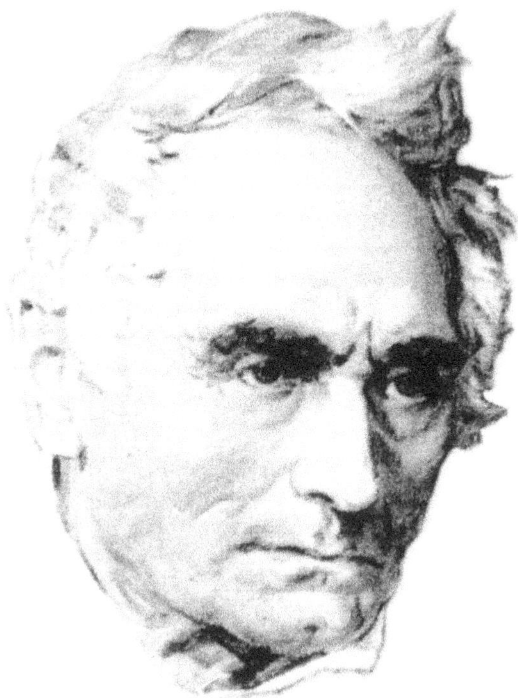

FIG. 3.5. Portrait of Purkinje, after a frontispiece illustration in Psotníčková (1955).

Beiträge
zur
Kenntniſs
des
Sehens
in subjectiver Hinsicht.

Von
Johann Purkinje
Candidaten der Medizin.

Prag, 1819.
Gedruckt bei Fr. Vetterl Edlen von Wildenbrunn erzbischöflichen Buchdrucker im Seminario Nro. 190.

Beobachtungen und Versuche
zur
Physiologie der Sinne
von
J. Purkinje,
Doctor der Medizin und Professor der Physiologie zu Breslau.

Erstes Bändchen.

Beiträge
zur
Kenntniss des Sehens
in
subjectiver Hinsicht.

Mit 1 Kupfertafel.
Zweite unveränderte Auflage.

Prag, 1823.
In Commission der J. G. Calve'schen Buchhandlung.

FIG. 4.1. Title pages of the first and the second editions of Purkinje's small volume on subjective visual phenomena.

4

Observations and Experiments on the Physiology of the Senses. Contributions to the Knowledge of Vision in its Subjective Aspect

A translation of Purkinje's first book on subjective visual phenomena is given in this chapter. As indicated on the title pages opposite, the book was published first in 1819 and then reprinted with a slightly longer title in 1823 and this version was included in the first volume of his *Opera Omnia* published in 1918, and in the *Opera Selecta* of 1948. The translation here is based on the reprinted editions of the book. All the figures were originally printed on a single plate at the end of the book (see Fig. 3.2) but they are presented here at the locations corresponding to the text describing them with the figure number for this chapter in [square] brackets following the original figure numbers.

It is surprising that a book defining an area of enquiry has not been translated into English. The surprise is even greater when one considers that Purkinje himself was considering having translations made in the 1820s. In a letter to J. Schmid, written in 1826, he wrote "I wanted to draft a concise overview of my existing work on subjective vision, and you were to prepare its translations into English and French, so that it would be better known in those countries" (Kruta, 1964b, p. 173). Unfortunately, the pressure of work prevented Purkinje from preparing the overview, and so the present translation might be considered as supplying that want. In his eighth decade Purkinje wrote "I have conceived a plan for continuing [the series] by a third volume entitled *Psychology of Vision* for which I still have copious handwritten materials" (Brožek & Hoskovec, 1987, p. 12), but this plan was not fulfilled.

The language in which the book was written poses certain problems for a translator. Purkinje's style was not always an example of clarity, in part because the important theoretical issues of his day were not necessarily ones that we now share, and in part because some of his sentence constructions were convoluted. Nonetheless, we have tried to make the meaning of the text accessible to a modern reader. Fortunately, Purkinje was principally concerned with his vision rather than with the theory of vision. However, because it was his subjective vision rather than his responses to external stimuli, there remain sections of text that we found difficult to interpret. In addition, some of the terms have either changed their meaning or are no longer used. Some units of measurement that he gave are no longer in vogue; where this has occurred we have given the modern equivalents in [square] parentheses. Even though Purkinje did not cite many references in his text we have not been able to locate all of them. The style in which the references are cited by Purkinje has been retained.

OBSERVATIONS AND EXPERIMENTS ON THE PHYSIOLOGY OF THE SENSES. BY J. PURKINJE CONTRIBUTIONS TO THE KNOWLEDGE OF VISION IN ITS SUBJECTIVE ASPECT.

Contents

I. Light and Shade Figures
II. Pressure Figures
III. Appearance of the Previous Figure under other Conditions. Clarification Experiment
IV. Galvanic Light Figures
V. Wandering Cloudy Stripes
VI. A Light Phenomenon in the Dark Field of My Right Eye During Increased Activity of the Left Eye
VII. Scintillating Light Points When Viewing a White Surface. Spontaneous Spots of Light in the Visual Field
VIII. The Place of Entry of the Optic Nerve
IX. Disappearance of Objects Outside the Entry of the Optic Nerve
X. The Entry Point of the Optic Nerve Visible as a Luminous Circle
XI. Appearance of Light at the Entry of the Optic Nerve
XII. Halos
XIII. Vascular Patterns of the Eye

XIV. Afterimages
XV. Cloudy Streaks While Viewing Parallel Lines
XVI. Zigzag Scintillations Following Observation of Parallel Lines
XVII. Changes of Parallel Straight Lines into Wavy Lines
XVIII. Voluntary Movement of the Pupil
XIX. A Spot in the Middle of the Visual Field During Strenuous Near Fixation
XX. Visibility of Blood Circulation in the Eye
XXI. Flying Gnats
XXII. Curvilinear Star Pattern
XXIII. A Pulsating Figure
XXIV. Luminous Rings
XXV. Unity of the Two Visual Fields. Double Vision
XXVI. Staring Vaguely into the Distance
XXVII. Eye Movements
XXVIII. Persisting Images, Imagination, and Visual Memory

When humans first develop self-consciousness the whole world of objects appears suspended like a dream. At first fantasy and dreams co-mingle delightfully; slowly, we become oriented in the circle of existence. However, something remains in the province of the senses and it cannot be transferred beyond the sphere of the individual.

There are sensations that do not correspond to anything outside the body. Insofar as they imitate the qualities and forms of external things, they thereby often give rise to illusions, phantoms, or appearances with no corresponding reality. These can be referred to as subjective sensory phenomena. Yet it remains the undeniable task of the natural scientist to establish their objective basis while for the general use it is enough to know that they involve only the sensory organs and that we need not search for external objects.

Several of these phenomena have become subjects of optics and, more recently, of the theory of colors. Although some have been incorporated into an existing branch of science, the majority have assumed a special pathology. However, from the standpoint of pure science there are as few pathological conditions as there are weeds for a botanist or rubbish for a chemist. These concepts are relative, and have validity only in so far as they remove a problem in reaching a specific goal.

The physiologist searches to find a law of nature manifested in the phenomena with the same interest as the apparent exceptions and complications, in the firm belief that they too reveal an all-pervading harmony.

Should we wish to place the study of subjective sensory phenomena into the overall system of sciences, it might be difficult to indicate its proper place, as each topic may be examined from many sides. In the first place it would fit into so-called empirical psychology. However, many sensory phenomena call for the study of material and dynamic relationships in the framework of an individual organism.

A rigorously conceived physiology deals with only objective phenomena and eliminates sensations altogether. For physiology, these constitute nothing but letters and words providing information about topics, the grammar of which is the subject of a special science.

Seen from a less rigid point of view, all of these border distinctions are arbitrary and their value consists primarily in the fact that they can be understood more comprehensively as special tendencies of the mind.

It would be more appropriate to place this subject, located at the very border of empirical knowledge, in descriptive natural science. Then there would be a natural science of the senses and a sensory realm in the confines of which the sensations could be placed in harmonious groups and considered in reference to a variety of relationships.

We can study, through observations and experiments, each sense independently as well as in its specific responses to the external environment. Each sense, in a way, is an individual organ. This is the reason for the specificity of the senses.

The only way to pursue research in this field is by rigorous sensory observation and experimentation on the individual organism. Both are important branches of natural sience in general and call for a specific direction of attention and a specific methodological sequence of discipline, training, and skill. These are subjects of research that can only be studied in this way otherwise they would not be accessible.

By these means the study of nature would add to both the objective and subjective spheres. The apparent disproportion of the magnitude of the two spheres should not mislead us, as the subjective sphere is just beginning to be tackled. Nevertheless, it promises insight into a rich field, once the competition will sufficiently increase among those who are capable of focusing on the special limitations of the senses, especially in pathological conditions, and the terminology necessary for mutual communication is created.

I have found several aspects of this that are new to me, or at least that I have pursued in greater detail than elsewhere. In the present work I will proceed by describing the conditions under which a sensory phenomena became known to me, together with stating their consequences. I will also draw attention to analogies between the separate phenomena, as well as between them and those of the external world, without wishing to pretend to provide successful explanations of them. Thus, I am convinced that we can only expect more complete solutions when we recognize the relation between each subject and the totality of its appearances.

For the moment I will restrict myself to the sense of sight.

I.
LIGHT AND SHADE FIGURES

The lively mind of the child revels in the manifold stimuli of the external world. It gives form to the vague, it rejoices in the repetition of what was done. Every moment brings a new discovery, brings newer and ever richer worlds of experience.

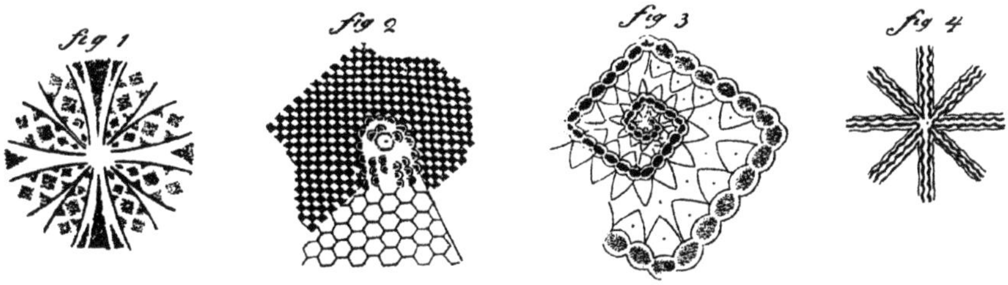

FIG. 4.2. Light and shadow figures (Figs. 1–4).

Above all they have pleasure in following the path of joyful light and immersion in the stimulating colors of the present.

Who does not remember, if only dimly, such games from that beautiful time? One of them, which could keep us busy at a more serious age, is as follows: I stand in bright sunlight with closed eyes and face the sun. Then I move my outstretched, somewhat separated, fingers up and down in front of the eyes, so that they are alternately illuminated and shaded. In addition to the uniform yellow–red that one expects with closed eyes, there appear beautiful regular figures that are initially difficult to define but slowly become clearer. When we continue to move the fingers, the figure becomes more complex and fills the whole visual field (Figs. 1–4.)[Fig. 4.2].

This is what happens in general. Now to the single instances and to closer definition of the conditions. I will first consider the observations of the figures in my right eye, and will mention those for the left eye later.

In general, I differentiate primary and secondary forms in the whole figure. The primary patterns define the background while the secondary are superimposed on it. The primary forms are larger and smaller squares (Fig. 2) alternately light and dark, which cover most of the field, resembling a chess board.

At the borders of the squares longer and shorter zigzag lines develop that appear here and there and then vanish. Outward from the center, which is marked by a dark point surrounded by a light area, I see a field of larger hexagons, with gray sides and white centers. To the lower left of the central spot I see overlapping half circles, the direction of which continuously changes. They resemble tree rings or roses with many petals.

In order to obtain a pattern not complicated by the secondary features, we should direct an open eye to a white surface, such as an evenly covered sky or a large white wall, and pass the outstretched fingers up and down in front of the eye.

The fine arcs of light in the center become particularly vivid when one looks from a near distance into the flickering flame of a candle. Furthermore, the checkerboard pattern appears fairly clearly when we view Newton's color disk rapidly rotating in a bright field. The disk does not need to be made in a standard way. It suffices when the number of white and black segments alternate. The narrower the segments, the slower the disk needs to be rotated. Also other colors can be used for these purposes, except that the darker and lighter colors must alternate. The pattern also appears in the spokes of a wheel turning against a light background. The basic general requirement is the rapid alternation of light and dark in the visual field; the greater the difference, the more vivid is the phenomenon.

The secondary patterns, seen with open eyes, are indistinct and they are correspondingly more distinct when the eyes are closed and observations are made in sunlight. In this case the primary effects subside. I differentiate two principal modifications of the latter: A spiraling rectangle and an eight-ray star.

At the beginning of the experiment before the eye is overstimulated by sunlight, immediately turn the eye, covered only by the eyelid, toward the sun, and move the fingers repeatedly as described. Both figures appear in a sharp contrast of light and shadow (Fig. 1). However, the ray figure stands out somewhat more; and the rectangle can be seen only with difficulty in the spaces between the single rays. When we continue to move the fingers and do so rapidly, a "rectangular spiral" appears independently (Fig. 3). It consists of several straight lines that grow in size. At their endpoints they form right angles and from the center they go first to the right and down and then to the left and up. Careful observation reveals multiple lines. In the center there is a dark line accompanied on both sides by bright bands marked off by the bright background of the whole figure. In the background, between the individual lines, there appear indistinct squares. At the edge of the rectangle we see a series of light spots with a dark periphery. The further we go from the center the more difficult it is to differentiate individual parts of the pattern. The pattern is within the eye itself and moves with it when we try to fixate some point outside the center.

Sometimes the eight-ray star appears in the field of vision before the spiraling rectangle, sometimes later. It consists of a few rods that cross in the center and thus create a star pattern (Fig. 4).

They are striated and bordered in a similar way to the previous figure. Among the lines that constitute the pattern the brightest one goes from the upper left to lower right and then one that crosses it at a right angle. In the others dark borders stand out. The outer ends of the lines become indistinct.

Above all it should be noted that the secondary patterns, while more distinct, are very variable. The rectangle may move, and it readily turns into a triangle and the lines cross at different places, run in different directions or in parallel, and form closed triangles or squares; soon the one in the middle band is lighter than the others. All of this may be reduced in the last analysis to the appearance of the primary squares.

After repetitive sequences of these effects they form different lines whose relation to one another gives the secondary figures. Nevertheless, the patterns that I saw before are more persistent. I am inclined to believe that other persons would see the patterns differently, depending on the synthesizing activity of the senses. This determines which sequence is perceived bound into a unity. When several sequences are spatially similar they are likely to be identified more easily. As painters have noted, if one has a vivid imagination any irregular stippled or striped surface comes to contain most lively patterns, be they beautiful or grotesque, according to the mood and external stimuli. Neither is the result solely of the imagination. The objective conditions also play a role. When they change, stimulus is given to different sensory activity. Further I must stress that the patterns I have described, especially the squares, have been seen by the majority of people with whom I have carried out the experiments, in so far as they can be communicated by verbal reports not accompanied by drawings.

They do not appear in particular individuals under particular organic conditions, but depend on the general conditions of the human organism or even on generally valid physical laws.

The patterns in my left eye, which is weak sighted, can only be seen incompletely. The primary patterns appear as curvilinear networks rather than as regular squares. The secondary patterns, however, are the same, only they are placed at opposite sides. Since I shall refer to them again, for the sake of brevity I shall refer to them as light-and-shade visual patterns.

II.
PRESSURE FIGURES

The next in this series of phenomena are the patterns generated by maintained pressure on the eyeball. They are generated in very similar ways and they differ primarily with regard to the external conditions, especially the source of the light that, in this case, is within the organism itself. This is unlike the previous phenomena where we considered the sources of light outside the organism.

If I apply gentle pressure with my fingertips to the cornea of my closed eye there first appears a broad luminous ring, which becomes increasingly visible, and is composed of small light and dark rectangles (Fig. 5)[Fig. 4.3], which run obliquely from below left to above right. The outermost boundary of the ring approximates a rounded rhombus standing upright on a corner. The circular-shaped gap in the center initially appears as dark as the outermost region. Gradually eight pale radiating lines become visible (Fig. 6) in which the rectangles in the area of the ring itself become even lighter, so that soon all the shaded parts disappear. Then in one or the other lower corner of the rhombus there appears a white shining spot with sharply bounded edges. The spot spreads out and eventually comes to occupy the whole area (Fig. 7).

In the bright space I can differentiate fine curved lines that originate in the extremities and run concentrically or cross each other and constantly flicker. The external edge of the rhombus has an orange color. At the moment the phenomenon is very marked; after a period of darkness, we can see another weakly shining ring that soon disappears.

If the pressure on the eye is released completely at the point of greatest clarity of the rhombus pattern, the shining rhombus goes through the same series of color

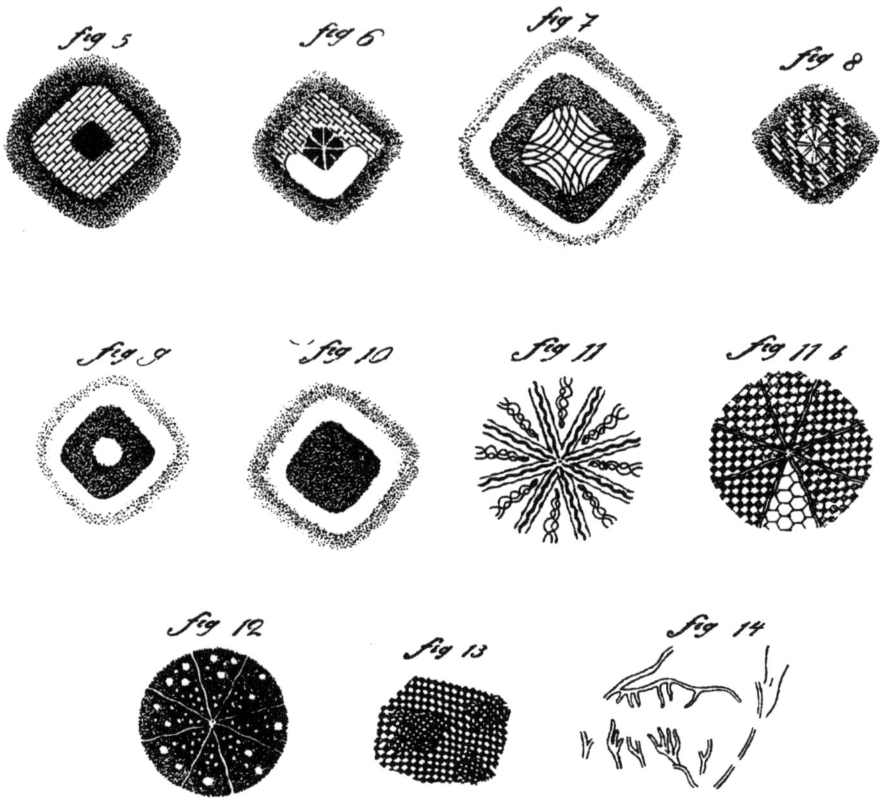

FIG. 4.3. Pressure figures (Figs. 5–14).

changes as an afterimage (No. XIV) generated in the eye by a strong external light (e.g., the flame of a candle). The luminous surface becomes narrower and a slightly violet border appears around the orange-colored rim that reaches inside while a bluish border moves outside. In both areas the squares appear again, but they are less distinct than at the outset.

The central area, surrounded by the ring, was also illuminated by a bluish, weak light, unclearly revealing those eight rays (Fig. 8.). For some time the area remains bright while the darkness that had surrounded the ring is replaced with a dim light. The ring itself becomes very dark. At this time, if we firmly close and then release the eyelids, the figure begins to return to its former intensity, only to disappear again in the same way. If we open the eyes at the time of the greatest brightness of the figure and turn toward illuminated objects, then these are visible only in the middle space and in the area outside the ring. The ring itself and the radii in the center either emit a weak light or, in the presence of a stronger external light, appear dark gray and half-transparent. In time they break down and individual dots and lines float in front of the eye in their place; they correspond to squares and radii. Usually I see several fragments of a blood-vessel pattern. When I close my eyes, they begin to shine, just like the dots and lines. It all ends with a dark rhombus with blunt corners, surrounded by a dull shine resembling a phosphorescent light. A total darkness follows (Fig. 10.).

During a uniform gentle pressure on the eyeball a different series of patterns may develop. At first one sees the pattern of eight radii in a gray light. Then the small squares and a rhombus with blunt corners appear. When the pressure is increased one sees a dazzling spot with two horns. It widens out until it covers the whole rhombus, but no ring is being formed. The disappearance of the figure is the same as in the previous case.

If, right from the beginning, I exert a strong and sustained pressure on the closed eye and continue the pressure, dim smoky lines can be seen on the whole darkened visual field; they go primarily from the center to the periphery, building mutually crisscrossing loops and nets interacting in a continuous alternation of light and dark (Fig. 11a). Larger and smaller areas covered with squares are seen between them (Fig. 11b) that slowly displace the earlier pattern and change into a shining rhombus. When the eye becomes confused through the repetition of this experiment, the serpentine lines turn into eight-ray stars and the small squares turn into a spiral of rectangles.

If the pressure on the eyeball is increased still further, a multitude of small dots are seen, first in the center, then in the rest of the space, forming rays (Fig. 12.).

They are bunched in the middle and disperse toward the periphery. Alternatively they appear and then disappear, always leaving a corresponding black dot that quickly fades away, only to be replaced with another point of light. Between these, more peripherally, larger circular spots appear shimmering in a bluish light; they alter in darkness but at a slower rate. If the pressure on the eyeball is continued, first the light points disappear, to be followed by the circular spots; only a few of the latter continue to glisten in a beautiful bluish light until these also disappear one after the other. Meanwhile an indefinite dim fluctuating light becomes increasingly visible; for a brief moment spots and rings appear in groups and rows that bump into one another; they consist of very small, regularly ordered little squares that move very rapidly.

However, these secondary patterns are not always irregular and dynamic. When the heavier pressure is evenly applied and the eye does not move, here and there stretches of larger hexagons can be seen (Fig. 13). Their touching sides are brighter, the inner part shines faintly and also consists of exceedingly small squares. If I move the eye only slightly or alter the pressure, then immediately the mutually dimming borderlines run over each other and a rapid surge runs through the whole pattern; this repeats itself more or less frequently until all becomes quiet and the hexagons reappear for a short time. Occasionally curved and dim streaks are visible in the center, and in some places outside the center, which rapidly move back and forth like the sails of a windmill.

If I release the pressure on the eye, bright branches and spikes appear (Fig. 14) like fragments of the vascular figure of the eye (No. XIII), eventually forming an obtuse rhombus, surrounded by a dark and then a dimly shining circle. In time its dazzling light outshines everything and then slowly turns into violet and blue and eventually disappears in the darkness.

Now I come to the related phenomena seen when the eyes are open in front of a light surface.

If the shining rhombus appears, and I turn the open eye to a clear sky, I see partially parallel and slanting, partially converging gray stripes; they begin to appear when the eyes are closed and correspond to the little squares and rays.

The visual field swarms with little squares and wavy lines when I apply strong pressure, and on opening the eye the daylight does not penetrate and the pattern remains unaltered. Soon, however, the pattern ruptures in the center and quickly opens on all the sides, with the dark area moving to the periphery and slowly disappearing. With even more persistent pressure the squares of the second order appear; sometimes it takes more than 20 seconds before the daylight starts to penetrate and for some time it remains clouded by the opaque fragments of the retinal figure and the converging lines and spots that all belong to the luminous rhombus with rounded corners.

In the morning, when the excitability of the eye is greatest, it often happens that a clearly shining retinal blood-vessel figure (No. XIII) is visible together with its origins in the entry of the optic nerve (Fig. 14). As soon as I release the pressure on the eyeball, the pattern breaks up in several places and the bright branches flow in curved lines and disappear like dying sparks of a burning paper. In general I must note that although I am able to excite the shining disk by so slight a pressure in the morning, I can rarely achieve this in the evening. By contrast, I can generate the checkered field with ease at any time of the day.

III.
APPEARANCE OF THE PREVIOUS FIGURE UNDER OTHER CONDITIONS. CLARIFICATION EXPERIMENT

Some circumstances under which similar cube figures appear now follow.

If I focus attention on a dark visual field shortly before falling asleep, I note, in addition to hazy stripes, to be described later (No. V), arrays of somewhat greater squares than those we have seen earlier that immediately pass through the visual field in different directions and soon disappear again. If by pressure on the carotids we reduce the blood supply to the head, there appear similar larger squares. Frequently we can even see a shining rhombus itself. We find the same thing distinctly during the onset of fainting. Also, during attacks of nervousness, the weakening of the nervous system in general, or following the use of narcotic substances, the cube figures appear during every strenuous movement or effort. Twice the shining rhombus appeared to me during heavy winter frost, without a feeling of discomfort in the remainder of the body. The little squares also appear in the visual field after prolonged deep breathing.

Finally, I also noticed the squares during galvanic stimulation when the discharges follow each other in rapid sequence, for example, when the discharge chains touch each other. However, in principle the condition may be reduced to a rapid change of light and darkness.

Now permit me to point out the analogy of these phenomena with others that occur naturally. As long as an observation of a natural phenomenon remains isolated, as long as it is not related to other more or less important experiences and applications (and by its impact on the rest of the system does not acquire significance), it is always in danger of being overlooked. Alternatively, if it did initially attract attention, it would soon be forgotten. Only when continuous development of knowledge points repeatedly to related phenomena does it attain the rank it deserves, so that it ceases to fall into obscurity.

The patterns appearing within the eye that I have described constantly bring back the memory of Chladni's sound figures and especially the primary figures. I distinguish between the primary and secondary forms of Chladni's figures. The primary patterns are generated by the moving parts of a sounding body, the secondary by the parts that remain at rest. It was the latter figures with which Chladni was principally concerned.

The primary sound patterns appear clearly when we place a layer of liquid on a horizontally held glass plate and then generate a tone by the stroke of a bow. Places that remain at rest in experiments with sand become covered alternately with beautiful raised and lowered forms of rectangular waves; they are smaller or larger depending on the height or depth of the tone, move toward one another in different directions, and create secondary figures at their boundaries where the liquid accumulates; in experiments with sand those grains ejected from the empty transparent spaces accumulate there.

This is an indispensable supplement to Chladni's experiments, and it actually brings us to the basis of the tones. Although Chladni's experiments with sand principally demonstrate the secondary lines, this experiment exposes the primary lines and suggests the origin of the secondary lines themselves. The experiment with the fluid becomes striking and exceptionally beautiful when we are able to generate particularly high tones. Then the whole surface teems with incredibly small squares that by the mutual boundaries between them create numerous and highly variable secondary lines.

The phenomenon becomes even more complex when several higher and lower tones sound simultaneously. Then greater and smaller waves run through each other in great diversity. These phenomena could be pursued further by measuring the tone waves, finding out their laws, studying the tones in more detail, and applying them to the physiology of hearing; they could be the topic of extensive treatises. I have touched on the subject only incidentally, in order to point out the analogy with visual patterns.

Now I shall present the train of my thought on these issues as it gradually developed.

After I have observed the tone waves many times, my active fantasy repeatedly attempted to relate them to other natural phenomena. Soon the world of tones did not appear to me in its deep darkness, but it was accompanied by delicate formations generated instantly by changeable waves, which arose quickly before my inner eye and quickly disappeared, exerting a lovely vegetation to the moving sea of air. What is lacking, I thought, is that these tone images are not related to the phenomena of vision in all their beauty. Only somewhat higher sensitivity to light, and tones will float in a multitude of forms before our eyes; because it is surely unquestionable that where so many oscillations, mutual contractions and expansions of a fluid exist, warmth and light, which always accompany each other, should also exist.

On the other hand, I endeavored to explain the visual patterns in different ways. I reduced the dry crystalline lens to fibers; observed the cells of a frozen vitreous body; microscopically examined the retina and the globules of its core. However, nowhere did I find explanation for the phenomena I have observed.

Finally I was struck by the similarity of the visual patterns of squares and the tone waves, and I tend to believe that both phenomena have identical objective grounds.

In general, where opposite, continually interacting forces limit one another, there arises an alternating victory of one force over the other with a temporal periodicity and spatial oscillation; the first one dominates the other at different times, the second dominates the other one at different places, so that in the apparent external peace there can occur substantial movement within and between the terminal points.

Thus, as this actually occurs during acoustic movement, so it appears to me to be probable that the eye, whether it is under pressure from the outside or contracted by its own force, enters into inner oscillation that lasts as long as the contraction; the contraction occurs to a different degree in all eye structures depending on their elasticity. The light that develops during these oscillations is in part within the nervous core of the eye itself and in part in the environment. The power of the senses generates the visual patterns that have been described. And so, as is usual, the tension, the magnitude of the oscillations, and the height of the tones rise and fall together. This also applies to the little squares. They can become very small when the pressure and tension increase, just as on the vibrating glass disk the acoustic waves become progressively smaller. In those cases where light and darkness alternate, to which the galvanic light phenomenon is, in part, to be added; I believe that as a result of stimulation and its absence an alternating contraction and relaxation in the eyeball takes place that generates an inner oscillation proportionate to the external pressure. Similarly I believe that we can think of a contraction of the eyeball in situations when the blood supply to the eye, as well as to the head as a whole, is reduced. This occurs because of the weakened activity of the heart, following the use of narcotic substances and during fainting, by pressure on the carotid veins, and by frequently repeated deep breathing; during these activities not only the brain but also the whole arterial system and with it soft tissues more or less collapse. Similarly, cold induces contraction of organic tissues; thus twice during severe winter cold I have seen the field of squares and the bright disk. I regard the shining fragments of blood vessels, which appear in larger and smaller groups and then die away, as contractions of the neural marrow, located under the central vein. As a link between the vitreous body and the retina it increases the pressure and with it the formation of the light. In a similar way I believe that the shining disk is generated by the crystalline lens. The sickle-shaped lines, appearing as tree rings and located in the middle, arise clearly from the lighter areas of the individual little squares. The larger hexagons are secondary.

The small sparks and the shining circular patches may be similar to electrical discharges that, as products of expansion and contraction, always reduce to circularity.

It is not easy to disentangle the chaos of phenomena that are being produced under the given conditions and to direct oneself to their diversity and inconstancy. I noticed them in my early youth, observed them as frequently as inclination and opportunity permitted, and, as the need arose to communicate the observations, I attempted to fixate them, record them by drawing, and express them in words. To be sure, others may be more skillful in being aware of the disposition of their system and its relation to consciousness. These experiments were in no way harmful to the eyes. It is possible that a lower responsiveness of the myopic eye played a role. Presbyopic eyes may require greater care in this regard.

The art of experimenting on subjective phenomena is in its infancy. Meanwhile the same rules apply as in therapy, which after all follows the same path; namely, starting at the lowest degree, observing the consequences, and progressing slowly to the point when the observed phenomenon does not change any more, or when we have reached the limit of sensation and there is a danger of the loss of consciousness, or when the sensation exceeds the tested range of endurance.

IV.
GALVANIC LIGHT FIGURES

Encouraged by the observations that were just reported, I was able to carry out a preliminary exercise involving the galvanic light phenomenon. I wished to learn if I could observe some particular configuration. As far as I could read about the subject, I did not find anything regarding the nature of this light. For my experiments I built a voltaic pile consisting of 20 pairs of plates (copper and zinc), with interpolated patches of cloth dipped in a solution of smelling salts. I used two guitar strings, covered with metal, as conductors. When I placed the conductor leading from the zinc pole into my mouth and touched the middle of my forehead with the copper pole, I saw in the middle of the visual field of both eyes, which were closed, a black curved stripe (Fig. 15)[Fig. 4.4]. Its concavity was directed upward

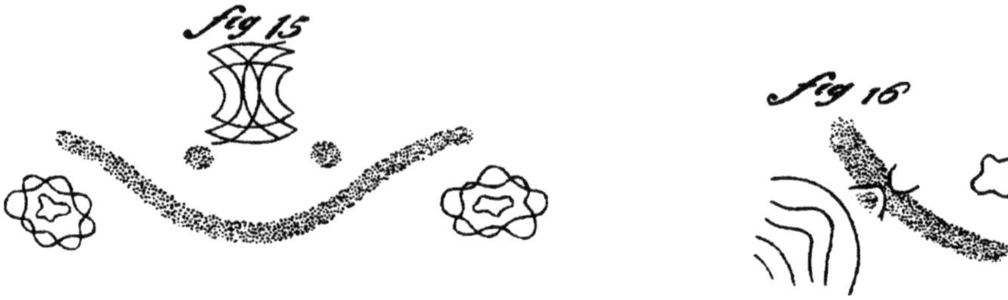

FIG. 4.4. Galvanic light phenomena (Figs. 15 and 16).

and the ends turned up and out; within the indistinct concavity and extending to the limits of an elliptical visual field was a violet light that was most intense in the middle of the dark arc. On both sides of this light and somewhat lower, one could see two sharply delineated dark spots that must be localized at the entry of the optic nerve. Under the dark band the visual field was filled with exactly the same soft violet light that appeared most clearly on the outside in the form of shining roses.

If I kept the right eye closed and directed the left eye to the daylight, the phenomenon became indistinct, then only one-half of the black bow could be seen, and the central part of the upper light coincided with the axis of the eye.

I exchanged the poles; then I took the conductor from the copper pole into my mouth and held the zinc pole in contact with the forehead; the appearance of the phenomenon remained unaltered, and only the soft violet light changed into a yellowish one. It weakly covered the darkness of the background and did so with the intensities reversed, so that the center of the visual field and the area under the external end of the dark curvature where the area, initially very light, was now very dark. On the other hand, the dark spot at the entry of the optic nerve was replaced with a soft violet, sharply delineated area that stood out more clearly, the weaker the remaining yellowish light.

This phenomenon not only demonstrates a light contrast in relation to the voltaic pile but within the eye itself the place where the nerve enters contrasts with the point of the axis of the eye and another point under the curvature.

Strangely enough, the position of the black arc changes according to the placement of the electrodes. If I move the electrode from the middle of the forehead downward onto the nose, then the inner end of the curvature turns down, whereas the outer end turns up. If I move the electrode on the lower eyelid from inside to outside, the curvature becomes unclear and appears to split. If I place the electrode on the outer corner of the eyelid, the curvature assumes a slanting position, close to the vertical, from below and outside to upward and inside (Fig. 16). Gradually it assumes a horizontal position as I return via the upper edge of the eye to the root of the nose. I could not tell what position the curvature assumes when I apply the electrode to other areas of the head or to the rest of the body. The phenomenon appears clearly only when I apply the electrode close to the eye.

When I change polarity quickly, as happens at every contact and its cessation, then I see waves of light above and below the dark curvature; they are parallel, alternately light and dark curved streaks that crisscross and create squares that are substantially larger than they were in the earlier experiments. Still better, they were visible when I touched the guitar strings against each other, without interrupting the electrode contact near the eye, and thus generated electrical discharges in a very rapid sequence.

If I applied pressure to the eye, the galvanic light phenomenon was displaced by the pressure figures, until under continued and increased pressure the retinal blood vessel figures appeared, which have yet to be described (No. XIII, Figs. 23 and 24). At each discharge, this figure appeared in the visual field in a strong, strikingly beautiful pale violet light at the entry point of the optic nerve. I was able to see greater parts of the figure than usual on the right and left.

In this case the checkered area can be reduced still further. Namely, it is formed by the crossing of parallel lighter and darker bands. The first are simpler, the second are compounded. Here we may consider the final structure of these phenomena. It would be feasible to formulate a general law according to which, in the context of light, tone, and crystallization, there appear secondary forms in the sequence of expansion and contraction; they penetrate each other in different directions and they can be broken down into their components (compare No. XXIII, no. 5, Fig. 29).

I wish to draw attention to the bent stripe that is there described and the half-moon patch that can be seen also in the galvanic figure (Fig. 16). I am inclined to place them and the firey rings in the same category with only a relative difference that in galvanically induced light phenomena a total contraction is initiated at opposite sides, in firey rings a one-sided compression takes place. The black stripe here corresponds to the black circle there.

V.
WANDERING CLOUDY STRIPES

When I fixate the darkness of an eye, well protected from all external light, sooner or later weakly emerging fine, hazy patterns begin to move. At first they are unsteady and shapeless, later they assume more definite shapes. The common feature is that they generate broad, more or less curved bands, with interpolated black intervals. These either move as concentric circles toward the center of the visual field, and disappear there, or break down and fracture as variable curvatures, or as curved radii circle around it (Figs. 17–19)[Fig. 4.5]. Their movement is slow, so that I usually need 8 seconds until such a band completes the journey and disappears completely. Even at the beginning of the observation the darkness is never complete. There is always some weak, chaotic light. It is strange that in this darkness the sense of proportions fails completely. The darkness is finite, extended in width. It is possible to measure it from the center, but one cannot determine precisely the peripheral

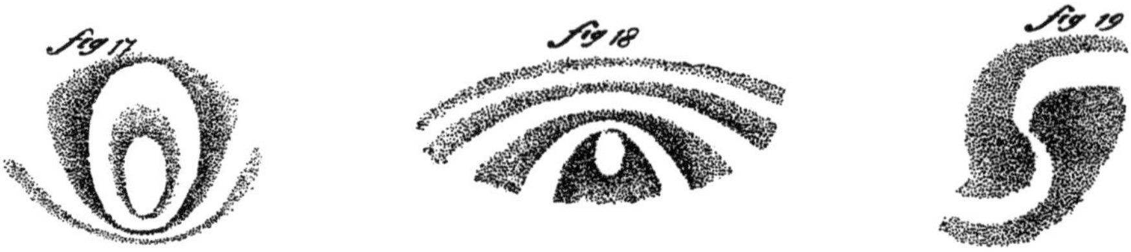

FIG. 4.5. Nebulous stripes (Figs. 17–19).

limit. The closer we come to the periphery, the more difficult and finally impossible it gets to establish a visible peripheral limit.

In order to clarify further the observations just noted, if I focused on all the effects, weak as they might be, after a few minutes light elements in the dark visual field in one case:

1. In the center I saw a weak light (Fig. 17), moving centripetally, that soon disappeared. Around it is a black ring, limited on the outside by a dim light. The ring also moves toward the center and the light is replaced with a black round patch. Around the patch a lighter ring is formed that is surrounded by a black wall that, in turn, is surrounded by a weak shimmer. Thus dark and light rings follow each other from the outside to the inside and are engulfed by the center point.
2. At other times the light descends from above as a broad horizontal streak of light (Fig. 18), the ends of which now turn up, now down, as the streak approaches the center. The parts of the streak combine into a single mass of light that once more moves toward the center and disappears in it. A similar but black streak follows the same path and eventually disappears as well. The same applies to light streaks that follow, etc. Frequently above the streaks I noted, when I was somewhat startled by a noise, some light and dark squares, so that the whole pattern was almost identical to that generated by galvanic stimulation, should the light be more intense, especially because its light is bluish and as a result of the color contrast the darkness becomes covered by a yellowish gauze.
3. Analogous to this are other cases in which the light and dark ribbons move from below upward or from one side obliquely and diagonally.
4. A different form of this phenomenon consists of two circling curved bands starting in the center and moving in opposite directions.

Later, when attention was reduced by fatigue, everything flowed in irregular waves of light and darkness, until even these straightened out and a hardly perceptible dim light quietly covered the darkness.

The figures described were seen with my right eye, because the left eye, which is somewhat weak, would not notice these delicate phenomena. In individuals in whom the two eyes are identical, probably the figures would unite just as the two fields of vision fuse into one.

These patterns point to those that were described earlier. If we imagine that bands of light come from several sides and move rapidly then they will develop into a field of loops and squares.

VI. A LIGHT PHENOMENON IN THE DARK FIELD OF MY RIGHT EYE DURING INCREASED ACTIVITY OF THE LEFT EYE

On a clear day when I have walked energetically outside and then enter a dark or at least substantially darkened room, a dull light flickers in the field of vision, similar to a dying flame of alcohol spread on a horizontal surface, or resembling weakly glimmering area smeared with phosphorus. On closer observation I note that the flickering mist consists of numerous very small irregular points of light that move in different curved lines. Now they accumulate in one place, create indistinct spots that separate, only to reassemble elsewhere. Each moving point leaves behind a track of light. The tracks create overlapping nets and little stars. Thus a large stretch inside the visual field swarms and impairs clear sight. This phenomenon is closest to the swirling of dust particles in sunlight.

The same happens when, having covered my right eye, and use my left eye which is weak and presbyopic, I fixate a light surface for a few minutes. A struggle develops between the visibility of the two visual fields and I cannot go on to focus on the visual field of the left eye. Repeatedly, the attention switches to the right eye, whenever the strength of will decreases. Its visual field moves like darkness in front of the object we wish to see. At that moment I am only aware of a swarming of tiny white dots, massed together and separated by a slightly black background, and they continue to whirl. The points appear primarily around the middle. To the outside they become more separated and irregular and resemble the previously described phenomenon. Finally, when viewed for some time with the left eye, they turn into a homogeneous flickering dim light.

This phenomenon is also visible when pressure on the left eye is steadily increased.

In all these cases the light points appear more vividly when the eyes are open than when they are closed, especially when one looks at a somewhat distant, not totally dark area. Therefore, in this case the external light is essential for the strengthening of the inner light. A more general prerequisite in both the last two cases is the heightened activity of the left eye, which brings into action the darkened right eye and stimulates active generation of an inner light. This may also have happened in the first case where my presbyopic left eye is looking into distance and is more engaged while the right eye is more or less resting. On the contrary, the left eye generates inner light that appears on a dark background.

VII. SCINTILLATING LIGHT POINTS WHEN VIEWING A WHITE SURFACE. SPONTANEOUS SPOTS OF LIGHT IN THE VISUAL FIELD

If we stare at a large bright surface, for example, at the sky evenly covered with clouds or a nearby candle flame, then in a few seconds light points leap up repeatedly in the middle of the visual field. Without changing their location, they again disappear and leave behind black points that vanish equally quickly. If, at the time that the light points spring up, I direct my eyes to a very dark place or close them, the phenomenon continues in a similar but diminished way, so that it appears at first view as if the points were ignited and then automatically ceased glowing. In order for a presbyopic individual to see this phenomenon, it is necessary to use a convex glass. Otherwise the distinctness of the external objects will deflect his attention from the observation of the subjective phenomena.

If one quickly closes the eye after seeing the bright surface before the light points have appeared, the points nevertheless form a dazzling structure that emerges in the dark visual field.

Similar, but larger and more luminous, points sometimes become visible individually, like meteors, even in darkness during normal vision. Suddenly they disappear and leave a spot that appears yellowish against a white background and impairs distinct vision. These are related to the spots that appear near a developing black cataract.

These phenomena, as well as the sparks that were mentioned in connection with the pressure figures (Fig. 12), appear to me analogous to electrical discharges in that they quickly arise and disappear, because of the conflict between contraction and expansion within the nervous substance, like those in the atmosphere.

VIII. THE PLACE OF ENTRY OF THE OPTIC NERVE

Marriotte's experiment on the disappearances of visual stimuli at a location in the visual field corresponding to the entry of the optic nerve is sufficiently well known, and has been clarified by Bernoulli and Euler with mathematical precision. I have repeated it frequently and thus direct my attention to the inner visual space of the eye. I must make note of it since I refer to it more than once.

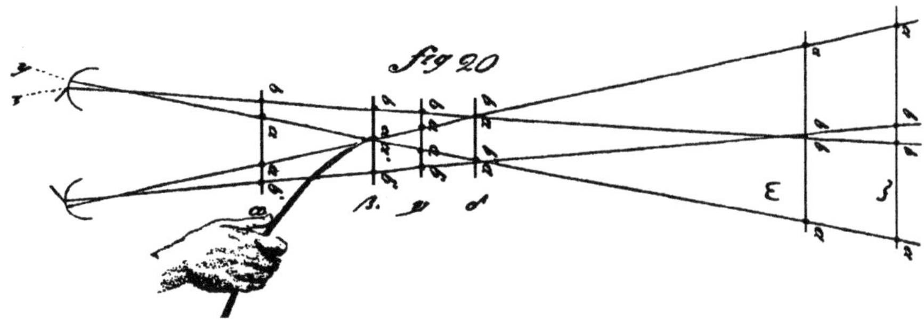

FIG. 4.6. The blind spot in binocular vision (Fig. 20).

It is easy to repeat the experiment in the following way. Using ink, we draw on paper two distinct points at a distance of 1 inch. The point to the right should be approximately one line below the horizontal. I move the face back 5 inches, close my left eye, and fixate on the left point. The point to the right will immediately disappear from the visual field, while other points, drawn further to the right, remain visible. The same, only with opposite sides, occurs with the left eye.

Should we wish to carry out the experiment with both eyes, we draw four points under identical conditions. In order to realize the whole experiment easily, we make four balls out of wax, place them on wires, and arrange them so that the balls are located in the relations just indicated (1 inch and 5 inches) and can be moved at will as the experiment requires. I identify the points that correspond to axial points of the eye (Fig. 20y)[Fig. 4.6] as *a* and *a'*, the entry of optic nerve as *z*, *b*, and *b'*.

Let us place *a* and *a'* at a distance that is shorter than the distance between both pupils (better less than an inch than more, in order to avoid making the experiment uncomfortable) and move a pin at *a* and *a'* to a point at which the left eye appears to meet *a*, the right eye *a'* (Fig. 20), where the axes of the eyes cross. Now we fixate on the tip of the pin, both eyes squinting slightly inward; immediately the points *a* and *a'* melt into one point and the two external points *b* and *b'* disappear. When one moves *b*, *a* and *a'*, *b'* (again 1 inch to 5 inches, according to the changed distance) so that *a* and *a'* overlap at a point in front of where the tip of the pin was (Fig. 20β) and we now fixate on *a*, *a'* as before with two eyes, then *bb'* disappear without any need for a pin. It is the same situation as before, except that the integration of *aa'* occurs by itself, without movement of the axes of the eyes.

When both eyes squint inward and the optic axes converge and cross at (*aa'*), the axes corresponding to entry of the optic nerve, in *bb'*, and the former with the latter cross in *ba'* and *b'a*. Now, with firmly held eyes, if the wax balls are moved by corresponding relative distances, as the figure indicates, into the crossing points of the lines, then each time *b* and *b'* disappear and *a* and *a'* appear in the visual field as a single point, while the balls assume now one, now another place in the tactile space (see Fig. 20).

In the case just referred to, if the convergence of the optic axes is fixated while the balls are being moved from one place to another, or conversely the balls may be kept on one and the same place while the crossing point of the optic axes falls either in front (aa' before $\gamma\delta\varepsilon\zeta$) or behind ($aa'$ after α) or between the balls. Then in the first case the balls will be located in the visual space as in γ or δ or ε or ζ, in the second case as in β (while a and a' may appear more or less separated), in the third case may be seen as a, b as well as $a'b'$.

To eliminate possible error, I must note that each eye can see the balls pertaining to the other eye, that is, in each of the cases referred to it is possible to see twice as many minus two.

With this I have traced a series of phenomena that, taken singly, might appear puzzling but seen together are clear. The last instance is identical with Picard's experiment noted in Smith's *Optik* (edited by Kästner). The reappearance and doubling of the central point (bb' in combination with e) by displacement of the finger covering points a and a' is readily explained by noting that the optic axes (y) do not pass through aa' as soon as the finger on which the eyes are fixated does not cover aa'. Therefore aa' falls outside the axis. Consequently, the points bb', which have a constant relationship to aa', leave the entry area of the optic nerve and must become visible.

IX.
DISAPPEARANCE OF OBJECTS OUTSIDE THE ENTRY OF THE OPTIC NERVE

Troxler (in *Ophthalmologischer Bibliothek* by Schmidt and Himly) also mentions instances in which defined figures in the field of vision may disappear. The general conditions are as follows: On a uniformly colored surface one makes a sufficiently conspicuous spot and around it, at smaller or larger distances, other spots. When we fixate the first spot (from near or from a greater distance, depending on whether everything is drawn in larger or smaller dimensions) and focus firmly for a shorter or longer time on the middle spot, then indistinct misty waves appear in the visual field, as on a cloudy day when the skies vary between bright and dull. At this time the individual spots or groups of them begin to disappear and again reappear. (Even the central spot and occasionally everything disappears, while the light background becomes only slightly clouded.)

During the very first experiment, the thought came to me that this phenomenon could be reduced to the wavy hazy bands described in No. V, and readily everything became clear to me. I distributed several pieces of paper evenly on a dark ground, removed any lighting from the side of the eye, and fixated on the central piece. After a short time the pieces of paper started to disappear. I waited until the effect reached its maximum, blew the papers away, and saw the well-known cloudy streaks appear in motion, wander around, and disappear in their usual way. This is related to the disappearance and reappearance of letters seen when one becomes sleepy while reading, because that is the best time to experience the cloudy circles.

X.
THE ENTRY POINT OF THE OPTIC NERVE VISIBLE AS A LUMINOUS CIRCLE

If I completely cover an eye and turn it quickly and forcefully toward the external corner, a large shining circle (Fig. 21)[Fig. 4.7] appears at the side. Its light flickers continuously while the inner space alternately becomes narrower and wider, as the eye, which is difficult to hold steady, tends to turn toward the inside and swing to and fro. This phenomenon is most vivid on waking. In addition, every time I suddenly turn the eye I see the whole visual field or only two curved areas located above and below, covered by large equidistant sparks that disappear as soon as a shining ring showed itself. If the visual field is illuminated, then the central area of the ring appears as gray on a white background. When the background appears red, with the light coming in through the closed eyelids, the color of the ring is dark blue. Otherwise, when the background is of a different but not contrasting color, the ring appears in the same, slightly darker, color. Around it the background is lighter (Fig. 22) and on the side of the center of the visual field there are minute stripes, alternately light and dark, that become shorter and shorter on the inside and here and there are broken. If, with the eyes turned sideways, one looks at the points *a′* and *b′*, then *b′* disappears in the ring. This adequately proves that it corresponds to the entry of the optic nerve.

Its light derives from the sudden stimulation of the optic nerve, generated by turning the eye to the outside, because the entry of the optic nerve is located on the opposite side. This stimulation generates electrical contrasts in the nerve and with them generation of light that expands into a larger or smaller part of the retina or is limited to the edge of the entry of the nerve; they are experienced in the area in which they are generated.

Should the idea, mentioned more than once, regarding the electrical discharge within the nerve substance and their visibility be correct, then we could gain

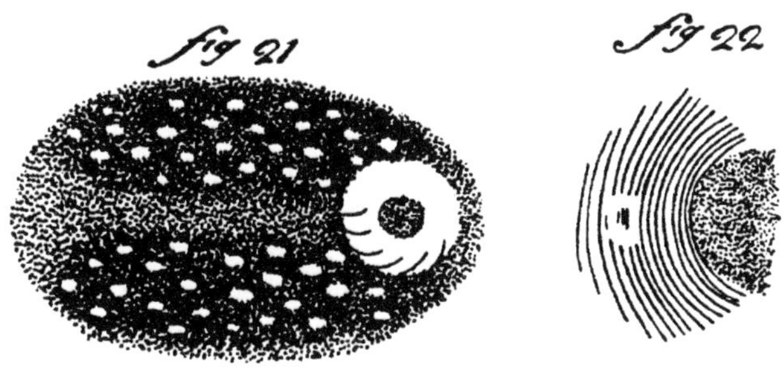

FIG. 4.7. The luminous circles around the optic disk (Figs. 21 and 22).

insight into the very core of the problem of electricity's spreading in space. It is in the nature of the sense of vision that what otherwise we are able to measure laboriously from place to place, we see fully at once. This was proved very well by Seebek's entoptic figures, the troublesome measuring of which was preceded by the measurement of singly and doubly refracting areas in the glass cube.

I must add that every time I was involved for some time with this experiment, I began to suffer from vertigo and nausea.

XI.
APPEARANCE OF LIGHT AT THE ENTRY OF THE OPTIC NERVE

As pointed out in section IX, Troxler correctly noted that the entry area of the optic nerve is not insensitive to light, as was believed earlier, because it always appears colored by the light of the background. Furthermore, it appears with a shining nimbus of light if, in lieu of the ordinary image, at an appropriate distance, we place a flame. This observation alone empirically refuted Mariotte's assertion that the choroid, onto which the images of objects are projected, is the proper organ of vision. Then how could an area at which no choroid is present be sensitive to light?

Rather it appears that the choroid does not account for light sensitivity but disperses light in the transparent medium, even in the retina, into indefiniteness and in this way makes possible the formation of the images. Where the choroid is absent, there will be sensitivity to light but no image will be formed. In order to examine the subject more closely, I took a burning wax taper (in order to make the flame as small as possible) and placed my outstretched hand at a place in the visual field corresponding to the location of the optic nerve. Immediately the flame disappeared and a nice red nimbus became visible in its place. The nimbus is perfectly regular. However, if one shifts the flame only slightly downward or upward to the outside, then a black hole appears on the opposite side that widens parabolically upward, downward, or sideways, and on the edges it is limited by the intensity of the flame. When I move the flame around in a small circle, the dark hole with light edges moves around in the opposite direction.

I find the greatest similarity in these movements of light and shadow to those that we encounter when a bead of an impure pane of glass is moved to and fro in front of a circumscribed light surface. Around the bead, at the side opposite to the light, a shadowy image appears, at the same side a light image, depending on how we move the pane in a circle around the light. In both cases the same objective conditions could be present. As the bead constitutes nothing but a small glass lens, the thread-like optic nerve entering the eye and then the retina represents a similar structure.

The redness of the nimbus is due to the fact that the light penetrating the nerve core in the half-transparent milieu becomes cloudy. In the same way the light appears red when we look at it through porcelain or several sheets of parchment.

XII.
HALOS

Subjective fields are visible around light flames, around other strongly illuminated images on a dark background, as well as the widening of a light image itself; these may be related to the previously mentioned nimbus. I consider the retina to be a turbid medium. The turbidity is due to the discontinuity of the small spheres of marrow. Although individually they are transparent, through multiple reflection on their surfaces they lessen the intensity of the penetrating light and change its quality so that it becomes colored and has many directions. Consequently, according to the laws that are valid outside the organism, in a haze floating in front of a light or in a white glass there now appears a clear light, now a light with colored edges. The only difference is that the modifications of the light are generated in the retina, exactly the place in which they are also experienced.

It is evident that such light halos can arise because of the turbidity of the other media of the eye. Accordingly, the pigment of the choroid of the eye and the choroid itself exert substantial influence on the limits, intensity, and quality of light perception. This is due to the fact that the light penetrating the retina is either attenuated by the dark pigment or it has greater energy if it is light colored. This will surely affect the reinforcement and change of the light sensation itself as well as the coloring and the illumination of the shadowy parts of the images. Accordingly the objects would appear to us very differently colored and lighted, should we be able to put ourselves into the visual system of other animal species.

XIII.
VASCULAR PATTERNS OF THE EYE

The halos that were just mentioned enabled me to discover a figure inside the eye that, on the basis of its conformation, I call a "vascular pattern." If I move a candle flame, held several inches away from my right eye, in different directions and even in a circle, there appears, through the diffusely illuminated light, a dark pattern of vessels (Fig. 23)[Fig. 4.8] that originates from the optic nerve and has two principal branches toward the top and bottom; they ramify and bend toward the center of the visual field. In the middle there is a circular dark patch that in differently incident light appears as a cavity. This is due to its doubling, as each part of the figure exhibits a dimly lit secondary figure that is only halfway separated from the shadowy figure. A similar retinal pattern also appears in my left eye but the middle of the spot is irregular (Fig. 24). At the point where the branches originate both vascular patterns exhibit a dark elongated perpendicular spot, surrounded by a bright light. As I have noted in connection with the genesis of the light–shade patterns, this figure appears to me when I turn my eye inward and let the light come in from the side. Furthermore, it happens in connection with the galvanic generation of light but also when I strongly compress the eye. In addition it can be

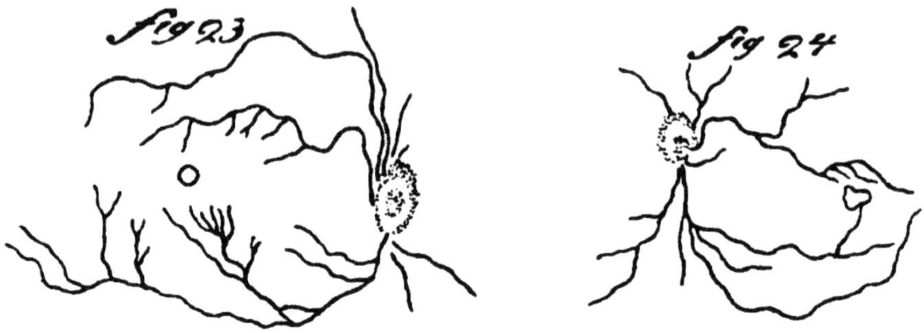

FIG. 4.8. The Purkinje tree. The pattern of the retinal blood vessels (Figs. 23 and 24).

seen in dim figures generated by afterimages. However, they are only fragmentary and appear briefly at twilight when I gaze for some time at a large white area and then quickly close the eyes.

Its form suggests that it is the image of the central vein, although so far I have been unable to observe any movement of blood.

XIV.
AFTERIMAGES

It is an imperative belief of the natural scientist that each and every modification of a subjective state in the sphere of the senses corresponds to an objective state. Surely the senses are the most delicate measures and tests of the corresponding qualities and relationships of matter. In the context of the organism we must examine the laws of the natural world just as the physicist is studying them in the external world using a variety of instruments.

Should the subjective realm penetrate all matter as intimately or even more intimately than it penetrates the nerve mass, we could probably discover a multitude of new, highly refined modifications of matter about which we have no idea. These may occur even if the subjective realm did not enter into a more intimate relation to the material realm. Where, on the other hand, this happens, a multitude of new and unusual phenomena must be apparent. They may be referred to as pathological because they disturb ordinary life. First of all this includes hypochondria and hysteria as well as a large number of other nervous diseases. Accordingly, it would be permissible to study the laws of light in phenomena occurring within the light organ itself, as we do in studying the phenomena of the external world.

As we seek and find in sensory organs what had been sought and found in the physical realm, we may anticipate and expect to find in the objective realm what had been sought and found in the sensory organ in the same way. In endeavoring to explain the pressure figures I assumed developments concerning light that exceed all the phenomena of the external world and are perceived only in the nerve mass itself. I believe that the same will apply during exposure to afterimages generated by a strong light or while looking at a strongly illuminated object. I have found modifications of the light principle for the images remaining within the eye, their variations and colors, to which no corresponding phenomenon has been found in the material realm outside the organism. Nevertheless, these phenomena are still material. I am inclined to believe that in each body, during and following illumination, a similar fading of light takes place, just as happens in the retina, even though it has not manifested itself so far. The sense of vision is destined to be finite. It would need to be infinitely extensive in order to be sensitive to all degrees of the factor that may affect it.

The glare figures or afterimages (as I shall call them for short, as in their nature they result from the blinding of the eyes) appear to be most closely analogous to phosphorescence. I intend to consider them in parallel, without attempting to explain one by the other.

On the contrary, they differ from each other. Namely, although yellowish-red light, just like white light, leaves vivid and long-lasting afterimages, blue light gives rise to weak and brief afterimages that do not pass through the sequence of red, blue, and gray, and then disappear, as do the former.

In the case of phosphorescence, we see just the opposite. Seebek's experiments demonstrate that blue light readily induces phosphorescence, whereas the yellowish-red color attenuates and extinguishes it just as quickly. Accordingly it would appear that phosphorescent light is related to a dazzling light like external to inner light. The yellow pole of light appears to dazzle and to irritate the eye by driving the light inside and accumulating it, whereas the blue light has a protective and soothing effect because it releases the light to the outside and thus relieves the eye.

Now a few words about the more precise development of the afterimages:

1. When I look at a flame of a candle only briefly and then quickly cover the eye with my hand so that the visual field is completely dark, then during the next moment there persists a similar bright image of the flame that is quickly extinguished from the periphery to the inside and is then replaced with a bright red image that in turn quickly disappears and leaves a dark space toward the center. During this time there remains the original outline of the flame in a weakly gray light that, after the first image has disappeared, slowly becomes nicely white and clearly represents the candle flame together with the wick. The phenomenon slowly diminishes toward the interior and leaves the original outline as a dark border, surrounded by a gray light.

Even when the white image has completely disappeared, only a black outline of the flame with a gray surround remains, until even this gray area decreases and becomes totally obscure. If in the first moment I quickly turn the eyes toward a white surface, for a brief moment the afterimage remains completely unchanged because the attention is fully immersed in the subjective sphere of the eye and because the external light is too weak to eclipse the inner dazzling light. However, as soon as the first moment has passed, in the darkness a white image of a flame seems to float on the paper that I hold in front of myself. It has a white border that in turn is surrounded by a weak shadow.

The grayer the objective background, the darker the image of the flame, until it again becomes white, in the same sequence as the background darkens. When I look at the flame for several seconds, the same changes take place but at longer intervals. On the average, after 1 second of viewing the flame, the afterimage lasts for 20 seconds.

2. The other extreme of this experiment involves a prolonged viewing of a candle flame. I have varied the period of observation from 12 seconds to a minute, and the duration of the afterimage is always the same proportion of the initial observation (1:20), as is the sequence of images of the flame, except that in this experiment the intensity and the duration of the colors predominate. In order to imagine the whole experience more easily and clearly, think about a dazzling white, a yellow, a red, a blue, a mild white, and a black flame image of the same size, and like leaves placed on top of and completely obscuring one another. In the first moment after observation of the light source, with the eyes covered, one sees the dazzling image of the flame, but it disappears very quickly from the outside inward, leaving the yellow; this lasts longer than the previous one, and disappears in a similar way; the same applies for each of the following until the black one, which lasts the longest. This lasts longer than the preceding one and disappears in the same way; this is true of each subsequent image down to the black one, which remains visible longest until even this is swallowed by a gray appearance that covers the whole phenomenon. However, we cannot imagine that a colored image of the flame waits until the preceding picture had disappeared. In reality, starting from the periphery, they recede in the sequence from glaring white to black, with decreasing speed, so that their borders overlap in substantial measure.

The whole phenomenon brings to mind the color game in which we are tempted to imagine several overlapping layers of color, of which the topmost disappears when the pressure is diminished and makes way for the next one. I could not verify whether afterimages projected from a black to a white background would change their colors according to the rule of contrast. The yellow afterimage becomes invisible and permits the red or gray to pass through, the red is replaced with violet, and the blue remains blue or becomes greenish as soon as the whole background becomes slightly yellow. The black border enables the white to pass through whereas the gray light covers the white background with a weak shadow.

Of course the overlapping flame images are described only for the sake of clarification.

My view on this subject is as follows. In relation to the external light the afterimage behaves as a cloudy medium that, however, has its own source of light. If it is projected on a white surface, it appears yellowish whereas the weak light of the afterimage itself becomes invisible as a result of fairly strong excitation of the retina by the light penetrating from the side. As soon as the external background slowly becomes dark, the afterimage gradually becomes visible until it becomes completely dark. The afterimage appears darkest when the intensity of the external light just equals the intensity of the inner light. At this point its appearance is impaired most markedly by the afterimage because the excitation of the remaining area of the retina is intense enough to make the weak light of the afterimage imperceptible.

In the second experiment the same would have happened except that in the center the clouding of the external light is so strong that the dim and gray inner light is visible over it. The red and the blue images dim the outer light less, and the red light appears somewhat violet through the admixture of darkness. The blue image turns somewhat green because the very weak clouding of the external light is yellowish. In addition, I must note that when we have observed a light flame for a long time, several subsequent color figures succeed each other that are brighter than the earlier ones. They follow each other rapidly, so that close attention is needed if we are to see them. Within the afterimage, both while we observe it and when it starts slowly to disappear, for a while the circular spot remains in the middle together with some fragments of retinal blood vessel figure (Fig. 23). They retain their color even if it is very faint.

3. If one looks briefly into the Sun or at a glossy piece of white paper held in the focus of a lens, a glaringly white image remains in a totally darkened visual field. It continues for quite a while, until the colored images appear, which follow each other very rapidly.

In the three cases just described, once we encounter the longest duration of a relatively weak white afterimage, there follow the colored and finally bright white ones. It remains to be shown under which conditions the black figure and the gray appearances last for a long time.

4. From the sequence of the whole phenomenon I immediately anticipated that it will also be experienced when I gaze at a less dazzling light than a candle flame. For this I chose a window that I fixated for 20 seconds, when the skies were gray. As soon as I covered the eyes with my hand, the glass panes appeared white to me and the frames were black. When the white squares disappeared and were replaced with black ones, the crossbars of the window gradually became white. In this way the phenomenon changed between light and darkness four or five times, until everything dissolved into a weak gray glimmer. This lasted for 5 minutes and even then, when I withdrew my hand from the eyes so that weak light penetrated the eyelids, the image of the window stood completely clearly, with dark panes and white window frames.

In this case the duration of the afterimage is substantially greater than one might expect on the basis of the intensity of the light and the indications of the earlier experiments. The situation is similar when we deal with pieces of paper on a black background. The dark afterimages maintain a gray appearance that alternately dissolves and assimilates the borders of the image. Then it becomes reconstituted and the image reappears. In the middle of the change from light to dark, all the spatial borders disappear, only to reappear with opposite illumination.

5. The color images and their contrasts also belong to this section. If the illumination is stronger, they even follow the same sequence of changes as an afterimage of the flame.

6. Newton's rotating color disk belongs in this category of afterimages.

A rotating piece of burning wood leaves a shining circle in the eye that covers the darkness of the background; in the same way each colored segment of the disk leaves a bright more or less circular area in the retina; this varies according to the intensity of its color. The covering is, however, never complete. Everything that moves rapidly, whether it resembles a line or a surface, appears half transparent and lets us see the light or dark background as more or less cloudy. This lies in the nature of afterimages that, to a lesser extent, never completely eliminates the reactivity to outside light. The same applies to the color disk; the less vivid color segments form the disks just as well as the more vivid ones and mutually overlap and penetrate each other. Therefore the resulting color is never a pure white but a gray that crosses into one or another primary color. Yet this gray is always lighter than could be expected from a sum of the light of all the colors, because the afterglow of the afterimages must be added.

The subjectivity of this phenomenon cannot be doubted, even without considering the evident analogy with the firey circles. It can be proved as follows. When we turn the head or move the eyeball in a circle with the same speed as that of the color disk, the colors do not mix because each segment retains the same relative place on the retina, as a result of the movement of the eye. The same thing happens when keeping the eyes closed, during turning, and then suddenly opening and closing them. We can differentiate the individual color sectors, though less distinctly, while during a brief opening of the eyes the afterimage could create only a small sector of the circle. In both cases the afterimage can not appear, because in order to be seen it requires a background different in color from that of the original. This happens only when the eye is at rest and it is the disk that is turning around.

During strong illumination if I look for a longer time at the rapidly revolving color disk, slowly a light–dark figure (section I) of an open eye appears more vividly and clearly than is typically seen. This fully corresponds to one of the principal conditions, namely, the rapid change of darkness and light in which the colors more or less resemble shadow and light.

7. Finally I must mention the shining rhombus that goes through the same variations as the afterimages. Likewise at the end it leaves a dark image with a light surround that alternates between light and shadow.

XV.
CLOUDY STREAKS WHILE VIEWING PARALLEL LINES

For some time I have noted an unclear glimmering when I looked steadily at a field of parallel lines precisely engraved on a copper plate. When I move the page forward or backward or around a central point, the vision reveals blurry streaks and the individual lines become undistinguishable. When the lines are horizontal, the streaks are also horizontal but somewhat irregular. The vertical lines remain vertical, whereas in a field of concentric lines the shadowy segments move in a circle. For a long time I was unable to interpret the phenomenon. For a while I was content to classify it as a fundamental phenomenon among the afterimages. I clarified it in the following way.

On bright white paper I drew several parallel stripes, one line wide at a distance of 1 line [1/10 of an inch or approximately 2 mm]. If I fixated any point in the white sector for a while and then looked quickly at the next black line, the white appeared to me whiter and the black appeared blacker. The reason is that the places on the retina corresponding to the black stripes were not stimulated and were more sensitive to the white light while the black afterimage of the white area helped to increase the darkness of the black stripe. When I now moved my eyes back to the white stripes, everything appeared faded. The black stripes as well as the white ones became more or less gray, and some time was needed before both appeared more clearly. During the second glance the white afterimage of the white stripes in front of a black background becomes more distinct, as happens when we cover the eye. At the places formerly covered by black stripes now white afterimages were being formed. They were stronger and more dazzling at the time of the second view because of the contrast between black and white. While the afterimages were being formed in this way, the objective images had become diffuse. With movement of the paper back and forth, the afterimages spread over the objective figures, and vice versa. Furthermore, by displaying the horizontal line, secondary stripes were formed, the direction of which was determined by the primary stripes.

Thus I believed that I have clarified the phenomenon. However, I could not overlook the fact that in dealing with copperplate engravings I did not need to stare at it and the stripes appeared on initial observation as soon as I moved the paper. I explored the phenomenon still further and quickly learned something else.

I took the same drawing of one-line-wide black stripes, drawn on a white background, placed them vertically before my eyes and looked at them while I slowly receded in a straight line. As long as the stripes were in the region of my clear vision (from 3 to 11 inches), the edges were seen distinctly. When I moved further back, the white stripes divided themselves into two parallel pictures and this was also true of the black ones. They moved over the principal images, located nearby so that white was covered by black and black by white. One was shining through yellowish, the other bluish. This took place at the distance of 15 inches.

When I moved to a distance of 18 inches, the neighboring secondary and primary images overlapped, so that now white was overlaid by black, black overlaid by white, and the original images appeared again in greater intensity. When the eyes were moved further back, these changes repeated themselves several times until the stripes could no longer be differentiated. When I used successively stronger and stronger concave spectacles I was able to increase the distance even further. This is an amplified form of the phenomenon observed when viewing the engraving.

The objective reasons are probably the overlapping cones of light lying behind the focus of the crystalline lens. Also it should be noted that secondary figures that occur here have the same property as afterimages, as white covered by black appears bluish and black covered by white looks yellowish. In the same way, the yellow and blue stripes by overlapping the secondary pictures yield violet and green. It is the retina where a secondary picture is outlined, still accessible to external objects, only with altered sensitivity.

Finally, the following phenomenon belongs here. When we hold a comb with fine teeth close to the eyes against a white surface, then we see between the individual weakly visible teeth very fine black and white lines, running in parallel, no matter in what position we place the teeth. Here a similar objective basis may exist, except that the cones of light, because of the closeness of the object to the focus on the retina, could overlap several times. Besides one may assume that the layers of the crystalline lens influence both phenomena.

XVI.
ZIGZAG SCINTILLATIONS FOLLOWING OBSERVATION OF PARALLEL LINES

If I fixate on the parallel lines of a sharply drawn engraving for 15 to 20 seconds and then close the eye, there appears in the same place a scintillation of undefined light and dark zigzag lines, which run like waves through one another and perpendicular to the previously fixated lines. This scintillation lasts for a slightly shorter time than the initial viewing. Slowly it becomes quieter and uniformly gray, until afterimages of the black and white stripes appear. If the black lines are thin and the white intervals are widely separated, then the afterimages appear immediately after the eyes are closed, without the scintillation.

The black stripes must be close to each other and of a width identical with the width of the white intervals. The same happens when we turn them toward a uniformly white or otherwise colored background instead of closing the eyes. Until now I have been unable to interpret this phenomenon, although I do not doubt that it constitutes a modification of the appearance of afterimages. The principal requirement is that the lines must be very close to each other. This fact is most likely to lead to the solution of the problem. It is probable that the scintillation may be due to the change of light and darkness of the afterimages and their appearance.

XVII.
CHANGES OF PARALLEL STRAIGHT LINES INTO WAVY LINES

During intense viewing of the parallel lines of an engraving, one observes an oscillation of the lines that on closer inspection involves some being closer together and others farther apart, so that the lines appear in the form of waves. The essence of this phenomenon involves in part perspective, in part afterimages.

In the central point of the visual field, the lines appear as more or less separated, and they approach each other at points more distant from the center. When the central point in the field of lines is moved around, at the more distant places the lines appear closer to each other and become more distant in the middle, whereas the corresponding afterimages retain their form and in many ways overlap and crisscross. This generates their movement and extensive bending, which gives them a wavy appearance.

XVIII.
VOLUNTARY MOVEMENT OF THE PUPIL

So far, with a few exceptions, we have considered that the movements of the pupil are involuntary. I was able to subordinate them to the will, in the following way.

When, looking through a double window, I fixed my sight alternately on two grains in the mass of the glass that stood in a straight line, one behind the other, I observed that one grain became indistinct. This was the more distant one when I focused on the nearer one, and the nearer one when I looked at the more distant grain. In order to be able to observe the movements of the eye at the same time, I took a glass plate with a grain in it and held it in front of a mirror, on which I also marked a point. If I moved the grain so that the point and the picture of the pupil in the mirror were in a straight line, one behind the other (but both being visible), and looked from one to the other, my pupil became wider when I looked at the more distant point and narrower when I looked at the nearer point.

I repeated these movements many times. I tried to carry them out without intermediary objects, and I was able to do so perfectly. I can now generate these movements without any specific object, just gazing into empty space.

XIX.
A SPOT IN THE MIDDLE OF THE VISUAL FIELD DURING STRENUOUS NEAR FIXATION

If I adjust my eyes in front of a bright white surface for looking at near distance, as if I wanted to look at something as near as possible, a white transparent circle with brownish, half-transparent indefinite surroundings appears in the middle of the field of vision. When I relax the eye, the spot disappears and the white surface at that place is whiter than elsewhere. If I assist the eye, by pressure exerted anywhere on the eyeball, for near vision, the spot becomes dark brown and nontransparent and its surrounding becomes light violet, while the white circle in the center remains. When the pressure on the eyeball is increased even more, there appears a brown

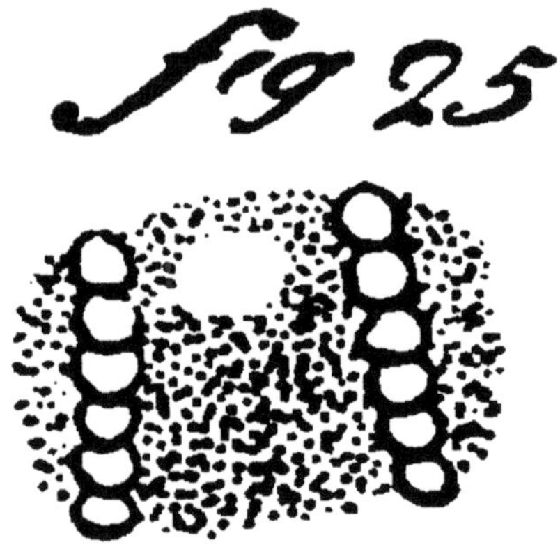

FIG. 4.9. Visibility of blood circulation in the eye (Fig. 25).

spot in the middle of the white circle or it disappears altogether and we see in its place some small white patches.

If I close the eye and keep it free from all external light, the spot is replaced with a weak glimmer of light, with a dark circle in the center. An individual unable to look intensely at a near distances may take a page of white paper and place it with one corner at the inner corner of the eye and now turn the eye forcefully toward the inside. In this way he will be able to observe more readily the phenomena just described.

XX.
VISIBILITY OF BLOOD CIRCULATION IN THE EYE

In the context of the previous experiment, for the first time I was able to see the blood circulation described by Steinbuch. In the dark spot on both sides of the white circle (Fig. 25)[Fig. 4.9], I saw two straight vertical light lines in which rows of blood corpuscles were moving, up to the left and down to the right. Once I became aware of the phenomenon I was able to observe the moving blood corpuscles using only a slight pressure.

XXI.
FLYING GNATS

A phenomenon deserves to be mentioned here that I was prepared to consider with the visibility of as blood corpuscles in the eye.

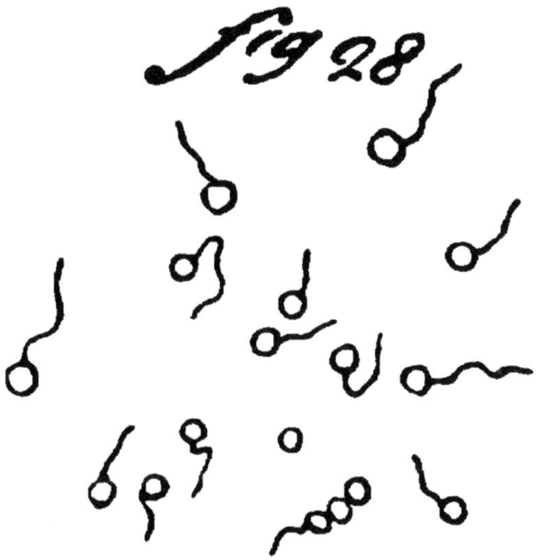

FIG. 4.10. Flying gnats (Fig. 28).

If during inflammation of the vascular system (either through physical exertion or fever) one stares fixedly at a bright white surface (like a uniformly covered sky or a snowfield) then many individual light spots (Fig. 28)[Fig. 4.10] suddenly appear in the visual field, which look like shooting stars in different locations, and move rapidly in curved and straight lines. When we view a restricted white surface, for example, a window, we note that each point, located away from the center of the visual field, is followed by a small shadow field.

Among the smaller fields I note some larger ones that are not easily visible; they look faded and move slower.

The larger ones can be seen quite distinctly when we are lifting something heavy, with the head bent down, or when we have made several violent jumps. They move like meteors from the outer limits of the visual field in straight or curved lines toward the center. On the side toward the middle they become light; on the opposite side they become dark. Toward the middle they become more and more faded and less visible. They can be seen only when the eyes are open and the illumination is appropriate. We must differentiate them from the light points, noted in No. VII, which are also visible in the dark and are of the same size. The fact that they require external light in order to be visible and are accompanied by a shadow indicates sufficiently that they are part of the body, whereas their external appearance and the fact that they appear more frequently when blood circulation is stimulated point to blood corpuscles. I believe that they are blood corpuscles swimming freely in a watery medium. At different distances from the crystalline lens they are larger or smaller and more or less visible. This determines their appearance and disappearance. This is even more probable because after

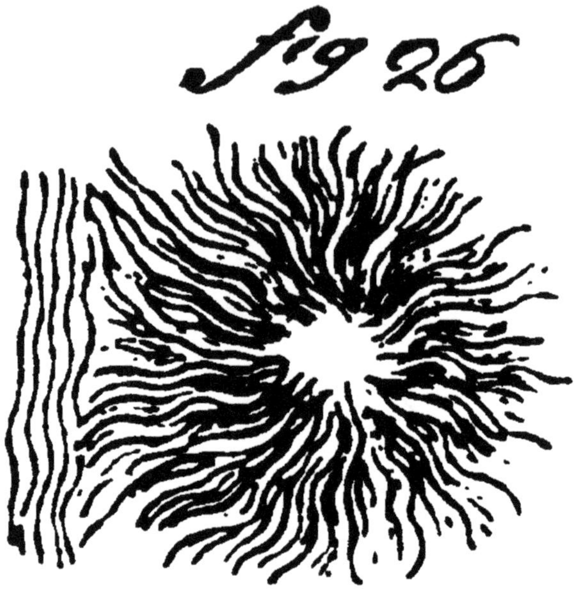

FIG. 4.11. Curvilinear radiations (Fig. 26).

bodily exertion, during which the venous blood is retained in the head, a sort of haemophthalmus may appear during which blood is in a watery medium. It appears to be more useful to refer to this phenomenon as "flying gnats" than as filaments and vessels that are visible in the vitreous humor. These never significantly change their location, whereas the gnats swim freely in the whole field of vision.

XXII.
CURVILINEAR STAR PATTERN

When I vigorously rub the eyelid against the cornea, exert pressure on one side of the eyeball, and then suddenly release the pressure, I see a small circle of light (Fig. 26)[Fig. 4.11] in the middle of the visual field. Outside of it bunches of parallel gray and white wavy lines are visible, now on this side now on that, depending on the location at which the pressure on the eyeball is applied. Finally, when the pressure is continued for some time, there appears the whole bundle of rays or a star pattern which on the right side is delimited by parallel vertical lines (Fig. 26).

This figure must be clearly differentiated from the figure described in No. XVIII and can be produced both with and without it. Because it is generated by the rubbing of the cornea, I believe that it is located in the cornea itself. The pressure and rubbing change the relative cohesion. In part because of change in light transmission, the different areas would be transparent to a different degree, although, on the other hand, the definiteness of the lines of the figure raises some doubts about it.

The figure could not be seen after being excessively irradiated by external light. On conclusion of this experiment, vision at any distance becomes indistinct for several minutes. The same happens when we gaze for a time with the eye resting on the elbows.

XXIII.
A PULSATING FIGURE

If I view the clear sky after running or other vigorous motion of the body (when the vascular systems are strongly stirred and the pulse can be felt in the whole body) I see groups of shaded gray and white spheres merging together (Fig. 27)[Fig. 4.12]. Two are on the right side of the field of vision, several on the lower side, three on the left side. They become more visible with each pulse beat and then disappear. They become even clearer when I exert pressure anywhere on the eyeball, where they become visible even without a preceding movement. The same happens during a fatiguing cough. Next to the spheres in the central area one can see a large circle on a white background that is slightly shaded. On the right side it borders on the arc of another circle.

Pulsating spheres appear on the periphery of this circle. A pulsating patch can be seen in the center of this circle; it appears when pressure is exerted at the side of the eyeball. Finally, during very strenuous coughing there appear several vascular patterns running from the periphery to the center of the circle. The vascular patterns are gray, white, and half transparent, and are even visible in a darkened visual field, emitting weak light. I regard the circle as an image of the crystalline lens in which the rays, falling in from the periphery because of a stronger reflection are weakened in their intensity (causing gray shading), whereas the light coming in from the side is less affected and creates a light circle.

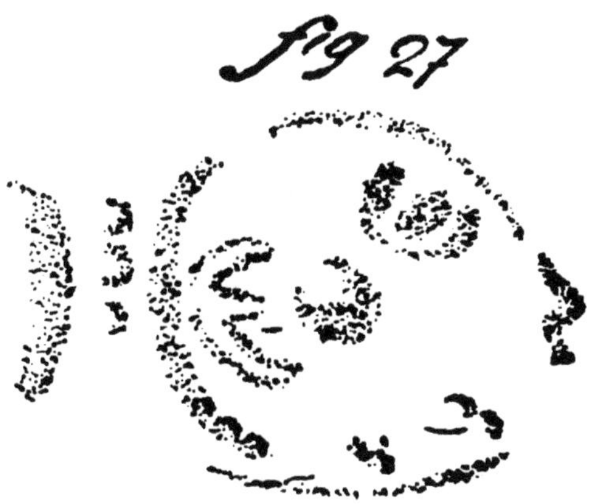

FIG. 4.12. Pulsating figure (Fig. 27).

I consider the pulsating vascular figures as the appearance of the central artery branching on the back wall of the crystalline capsule.

XXIV.
LUMINOUS RINGS

Eichel (1774) and Elliot (1785) observed and described the luminous rings that appear at the outer limits of the visual field. Eichel drew from it relevant consequences for the theory of vision. I found it necessary to observe them more closely in order to examine their relationship to other phenomena.

1. If I focused the eyes for seeing at near distance, the slightest contact brought forth the rings; however, in looking into the distance, the pressure needed to be increased substantially. This fact, and the appearance of a brownish spot for near vision, as well as by pressure on the eyeball, prove sufficiently that during near vision the eye contracts whereas it relaxes for distant vision. Home came to the same idea when he measured the convexity of the cornea during far and near vision. In the second case the unsteadiness indicates the presence of muscular effort.

2. These rings, as well as those described in No. X, appear at the entry point of the optic nerve most vividly after waking in the morning. They appear to be identical in their nature, they differ in only their direction; here the retina is pulled to the inside, there to the outside by means of the optic nerve. Analogical phenomena would have to take place if it were possible to pull the sclera to the outside at some place.

3. If we hold a quarter of a page of white paper at the inner corner of the eye, turn the eye forcefully inward, and then press toward the inside a blunt pointed piece of wood at the outer side of the eyeball, there appear in parallel (Fig. 29)[Fig. 4.13]

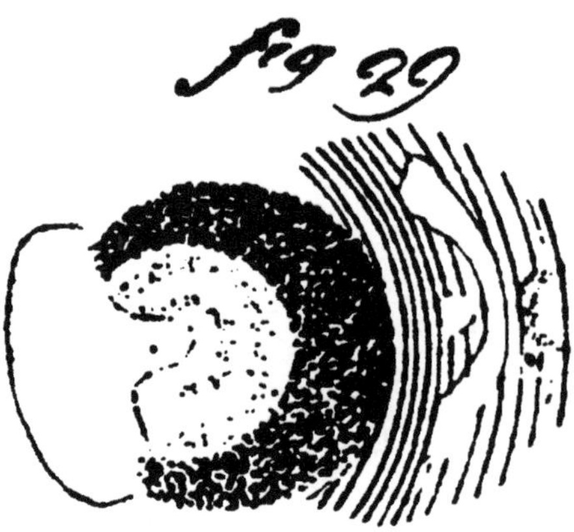

FIG. 4.13. Firey rings (Fig. 29).

many concentric, alternately black and white lines, as in Fig. 22 of No. X. They spread from the outer limits of the circle over the spot in the middle of the field of vision. If we change the place at which the pressure is applied, the black circles remain parallel. In order to see them really distinctly, we must exert pressure with the blunt stick as far as possible vertically into the space between the eyeball and the border of the eye socket. In this way the pressure reaches more deeply into the back wall of the eyeball.

4. By exerting pressure at the external corner of the eye in the way specified, one sees a large black, more or less circular spot at the opposite side on the white paper held before us. The parallel white and black lines appear on its side that is directed toward the center of the visual field. The opposite edge of the spot is marked by yellowish white light. If the pressure exerted by the wooden stick is increased, the spot first widens toward the center and then splits into two parts. At the periphery the spot is dark black; toward the inside it is dark green but also scintillating dark violet. When the eyes are well covered, there appears a slightly glittering black light. With justice, Elliot compares it to the eye on a peacock feather. In it we note in various areas the previously described vascular figure, black in the opalescent light of the eye on the peacock feather. The figure has the same ramifications as had been indicated.

5. If we exert the pressure far toward the back, so that the parallel stripes reach the middle of the visual field, we can see two white bands. They broaden to the outside, forming an obtuse angle and between them leave a small spot of light. On the other side where they join there is a brownish spot in the form of a half moon. Both follow each movement of the peacock eye while they turn around the center of the visual field as its axis. When the pressure is increased, the black spot advances to the middle, swallows the ends of the bands up to the point at which they join, which now appears as a white circular spot.

The half-moon spot opens up, moves back, and disappears in the parallel lines that lie behind it while a half-circular projection of the remaining light penetrates the area. The same bands and spots appear in the dark central strip of the galvanic figure, when we move the eye in the same way back and forth (Fig. 16).

6. When the pressure on the side of the eyeball is suddenly reduced, the white circular spot moves equally quickly back to the outside. For a short time it is replaced with a slightly brown and violet fog, divided by a white stripe into two equal parts. Usually the upper part appears to be stronger and darker than the lower one. At times in the center the stripe persists, especially in the middle, and impairs clear vision.

7. We can use this experiment also to convince ourselves that the visual fields of the two eyes combine into one. Namely, when we exert pressure on the corresponding area of the right and left eyeball, then the luminous rings are generated by this overlap. Having tested the effect of pressure in this way at all points that could be reached, we can measure the visual field in all its directions. By this means we can establish that each eye has its own visual field but that they fully overlap.

8. The scintillating colors described above can be seen in a darkened field of vision; they glisten in the middle of the circular patch, as well as the outer edge

surrounding the black ring. The concentric lines cannot be differentiated and yield only a dim gleam. When the pressure is released rapidly, a clear strip of light, similar to a flash of lightning, moves from inside to the outside. The yellow–white stripe, visible on the outer edge of the circular patch when the eyes are open, seems black when the eyes are covered and reaches just the middle of the patch. Initially it is transparent and then black, because of the absence of the external light. On the contrary, the blackness of the edge and of the concentric lines is a genuine sensation and asserts itself against the external light.

9. The following phenomenon is also relevant. If when I am washing my face the palm of my hand slips from the upper edge of the orbital cavity on the eyeball, every time a large light circular area appears to me in which the light is more intense on the periphery and weaker in the direction toward the inside. I note the same thing following a gentle sudden blow of the finger against the cornea.

XXV.
UNITY OF THE TWO VISUAL FIELDS. DOUBLE VISION

Just in the preceding section I described the way in which by means of firey circles one can demonstrate the mutual overlap of the two visual fields. One can do the same in the following way: Let us mark off the distance between the pupils of the two eyes on a sheet of cardboard and make openings on the two marked places. If we hold the paper tight against the eyes and look into the distance through the corresponding openings, then the two openings become one. The same happens when instead of the openings we make two black dots. These points correspond to the midpoints of the two visual fields. The two points, although 2.5 inches distant, merge into one as do the visual fields.

Now the thought came to me that the points could merge even if the distance between the two eyes was greater and the direction of the pupils was altered, for example, when they do not lie at the same level, as may be true of animal eyes. Therefore I took a page, bent somewhat its edge vertically, and I cut the bent part in the center so that I could bend it around the base of the nose. On this border, the edge of which was turned to the outside, at a distance between the two pupils I marked two black points. When I moved the border nearer the eye and looked straight into the distance, the two points were united in a single point. If I held the paper secured in the same position and pressed the index fingers, coming from above and from the side of the forehead so that both eyes were turned from the inside to the outside, and in this way the axes of the two eyes separated, the left point moved to the right over the right point and this one moved in the opposite direction for about four to five lines [approximately 10 mm] from each other.

If next to these points, at a distance of four to five lines, I drew two additional points, they merged again into one point. One may assume that with a greater separation of the eyes, should such be possible, the same thing would have to happen, as in both cases only a quantitative difference exists. Then even in the presence of diverging axes of the eyes, the visual fields would merge.

When we look at an object from the distance of a few steps and push the eyeballs apart, the image in the right eye moves to the left and the image of the left eye moves to the right, whereas in the middle between the two a pulsating patch appears, which regularly is visible during pressure on the eye and corresponds to the center of the retina. Should there, in the presence of diverging visual axes of the eyes, arise two fields of vision, then the seen object would have to move in the same direction as the eye.

Thus not only when the two visual axes unite at their ends but even without this the visual fields merge into one.

I conceive a possible reason for seeing this phenomenon in the following way. As long as our consciousness is fully immersed in a specific activity, each eye can be regarded as a separate entity; in relation to the external world each eye differentiates up and down and left and right. The same applies to touch. However, all these concepts are relative and they apply to the subject and its spatial relations to the object. Because there exists only one consciousness that unifies the separate individualities of the senses, so all the separate relations must merge into one. The same would have to happen when several human individuals could be joined into a single higher entity. On the other hand, there could exist a sort of double vision. Without altered spatial relations of the organs, it would be regarded as a mental illness, as a disintegration of the unity by consciousness into subordinated spheres.

1. If a single eye loses its individuality with reference to the total consciousness, so that what is in front of each eye fails to become unified, this does not take place in relation to the objects that lie on this or that side of the midpoint of the visual field. What lies to the right of the visual axis for one eye lies to the left for the other, and vice versa. The same applies to up and down. The objects lying between the two visual axes must always be seen double, even when the centers of the visual field coincide. This double vision will not be present when the objects are distant, as their relations to the eyes and the size of the visual angle remain essentially the same because of the great distance and the small visual angle. This does not apply to near distances, where the relations of a given point external to the eyes is of greater significance the more important the distance between the two eyes in relation to other distances. Double vision is particularly striking when both visual axes cross closely in front of the nose, for example, when one looks at a finger held before the eyes. In this case the visual axes diverge markedly behind the crossing point and many objects are seen by one eye as located to the right and by the other eye as located to the left. When the visual fields are united, they doubly overlap.

Double vision corresponds then to the nature of the sense and we are less aware of it because our attention is always focused on the merging axis points. In addition, one eye is frequently weaker than the other one. Thus the eye has a kind of abstracting capacity according to which it is able to focus on the sphere of one and then of the other eye.

2. Furthermore, there is another kind of seeing double involving only one eye. If one applies a gentle pressure just above or below the cornea, the images of objects become smaller and clearer. Depending on the pressure, faint secondary images appear on one or the other side. The same thing happens when one pulls the external corner of the eye toward the outside. Several times this double vision lasted for several hours after I had placed a small bag of iron filings on the eyeball overnight. I believe that this phenomenon may be related to the recent experiments by physicists according to which substances that normally refract light singly refract doubly under pressure and tension (Brewster).

3. Finally this is the place to mention the multiplication of objects encountered in nearsighted individuals when objects recede from the point of clear vision. If I walk slowly away from a book, beyond the distance of clear vision, at first the individual letters become blurred, while the secondary images run across the primary images. When the distance is increased, the same happens with the lines, as I described it earlier in No. XV when I wrote about parallel lines. It may be that the eyes of nearsighted individuals are overstrained and for this reason are doubly refracted. By an incision in the cornea, releasing some fluid, the excessive stretching is eliminated and the cornea again refracts light singly.

XXVI.
STARING VAGUELY INTO THE DISTANCE

Staring vaguely into the distance is a condition opposite to fixating on something and to strenuous pursuit of moving bodies or of motionless lines. Whereas in the latter case attention is focused virtually on a single point, in the former case it covers the whole visual field and gains in extension what it lost in intensity. This way of viewing is evoked either intentionally when we look into infinity with the visual axes parallel, as if we wanted to look through the intermediary objects; it also occurs unintentionally when we are immersed in thought with the eyes open or when our consciousness slackens or our thinking loses direction (especially during so-called emptiness of the head) when we are distracted, sleepy or dull witted. In these cases it takes a lot of effort to fixate on a particular object, and no sooner is this achieved than the fixation point dissolves in indefiniteness. The visual axes do not converge at a definite point nor is the eye engaged in activity through which it becomes able to see clearly nearer and more distant objects. Therefore the objects, located at a distance at which we normally see clearly, are seen indistinctly and the pupil is wide open, as in narcosis or in continuing sleepiness after we have been suddenly awakened. Both circumstances may well belong in this context.

The eyes are in the same condition when we want to be aware of what is happening peripherally without looking at it directly. The eyes are set for seeing ahead in the distance but imperceptibly oscillating in order to offer ever newer areas on the retina for the light coming in from the observed objects. Outside its center the sensitivity of the retina is readily exhausted so that all light qualities and contours become indistinguishable.

However, one must note that during staring the afterimages are imprinted more deeply and more enduringly than when the eyes are steady or move. This would follow from the rule that while thinking we should close the eyes and while in rapid writing or reading we should look quickly but decisively at every line of what is being written or what is to be read rather than being satisfied with general impressions made by individual characters and words.

XXVII. EYE MOVEMENTS

First it is necessary to refer to the movements by which the center of the field of vision, where seeing is clearest, follows the boundaries and lines of external objects. When dealing with small objects, such as features of letters, even superficial attention enables us to follow these patterns with our eyes; this is easier if the objects are larger. Such perception permits us to be aware of the different degrees and directions of tension in the eye socket. Extreme tension is generated during vigorous rotation of the eyes. When we pay attention to these tensions, with the head held steady, and pursue various straight and curved lines, we find that it is not equally easy to follow different figures. We can follow circular patterns most readily. Straight lines, no matter what their direction, are more difficult to follow. It appears that we have to apply force in order to keep the eye from deviating to the side when the eye passes through the center of the visual field. As regards straight lines, it is easiest to follow horizontal and especially vertical lines. This proves that habit and exercise exert important influence, as it is these lines that we see most frequently in daily life.

The fact that it is easier for the eye to follow the circumference of a circle is due to the tendency toward equilibrium of the antagonistic eye muscles. This tendency is similar to the centripetal force that continues at all times to steer the movement in a straight line from the periphery toward the center, without requiring one's own voluntary effort. Similarly, it is easier for the eye to move toward the external corner of the eye downward than upward, because of the place at which the optic nerve enters the eyeball and its greater or smaller pull; this takes place during the movements that have been mentioned. The pull is greater when the movement is directed outward and upward, which can bring about pain and a kind of daze. In the presence of sharp pain, this movement is carried out instinctively, as if one wanted to reduce one pain by another or by numbing.

When we look at regular geometric figures—spirals, circles, and wavy lines, symmetrical patterns, ornaments, and decorations—where order and necessity rule, the eye feels as if it is being pulled away from the outlines of the objects.

The movements are easier, half automatic, so that they are transferred to the objects at which we are looking and that seem to manifest their own life and movement. This makes a strange impression and is also accompanied by sensations of tension in the eyeball. It would be worth the effort to define this kind of optic music as a separate art form, which beckons to us everywhere in nature and in the world of art. Surely this would open a new path for a creative genius, if the implementations were of sufficient magnitude. As of now the time for this art does not seem to have arrived. It must serve as a slave to the adornment of clothes, buildings, and gardens. Only in fireworks, dance and gymnastic performances, altars, flower gardens, transparent circles with movements in the center, and as of late in the kaleidoscope did this art take on an independent life. However, because it marches through the world jointly with clowns, it is unrecognized by aristocratic taste and is overlooked.

When we observe ourselves in a quiet, inwardly directed thought, in darkness or with the eyes closed, we become aware of delicate movements of the eyes, which probably accompany visual images. The eye also has its sense of touch, and one could argue that touch is better developed in the eyes than in any other organ of movement. The movements of the eye in blind people are probably nothing other than the activity of the sense of touch, which either accompanies thought or reduces the images of the sense of touch of the hands into a smaller, more readily manageable scale. Therefore the eyes of the blind individuals express mental processes, even though we might be tempted to presume that the expression of the eyes would be totally lifeless because of the absence of vision. Although these eye movements are so rapid and so short that they would be hardly perceptible to another person, nevertheless it is my view that they constitute the very essence of a human condition. The direction of gaze is either wandering and aimless (as we encounter in the insane), or dull and vague (as in the feeble minded), fresh and lively or slow and staring, quiet, moving rhythmically with a comprehension of individual features, wild or gentle, strong, weak, lost in looking at something, spirited or dull. The infinite number of its modifications constitutes a most interesting language that can be comprehended by only a refined sense for physiognomy.

During perfect vision, the focus moves through all the meeting points and lines of an object. During superficial vision only some points and lines are noted, whereas the remaining ones are overlooked or only indistinctly perceived from the side. Well-known details are enriched by imagination.

It would be an important subject of pedagogical methodology to provide firm and necessary rules for the perceptual activity of the eye. Only then can appropriate training begin that can lead to virtuosity—the highest aim of all education.

XXVIII. PERSISTING IMAGES, IMAGINATION, AND VISUAL MEMORY

I have frequently been surprised that blinking the eyes does not disturb vision, as I imagine that total darkness must occur during blinking. On closer observation, however, I established that the visual field of the open eyes, with all its lights and images, persists for a while after closing the eyelids. The more attentively I look at a simple, not too extensive image, the longer I can maintain it in my mind after I have closed my eyes. This persisting image must be rigorously differentiated from afterimages. The mental image can be maintained for a longer time only by the action of the mind and disappears as soon as the will slackens. It can, however, be brought back voluntarily. On the other hand, the afterimage floats involuntarily before the eyes, disappears, and reappears as a result of objective facts.

The spatial activity of the eye, the sense of feeling of the eye, projects the persisting image outside the eye itself, just as happens during actual seeing. It can also represent stereometrically limited images and the memory image even maintains its original location and position during the movement and turning of the whole body. By contrast, the afterimage represents only surfaces; it is located in the eye and follows its movements. The vividness of the memory image differs according to the differences in mood. It is particularly vivid in the presence of a more intense mental activity following the consumption of alcoholic beverages or narcotics or when one is interested in a particular object. In the presence of feverish excitement of the blood, especially in the presence of cerebral affectations, it rises to the level of hard objectivity.

The afterimage, on the other hand, is likely to persist longer in the presence of nervousness and asthenia. It disappears faster the livelier the activity of the eye. Furthermore, the memory image is more distinct and objective the closer we are to the moment during which the pattern was originally perceived. During each moment that follows, it is gradually more difficult to keep the image clear. On the contrary, the afterimages of weakly glowing objects, in the first moments after they had been seen are unclear and develop only slowly while we remain passive onlookers.

I believe that through practice, while we are able to maintain the image longer and more closely after the initial perception of an object, the image could approach the realism of the original perception. This practice might be important for the training of memory and imagination.

One could ask in which organ the persisting image is located. As regards the original image and the afterimage, it is widely believed that they are experienced in the retina. With equal justification one could maintain the same view regarding the persisting image. The empirical evidence in both cases is compelling.

According to this point of view, one could maintain that memory and imagination could be active in the sensory organs themselves and that each sense possesses a specific memory and imagination. As limited forces they are subordinated to the general mind.

The primary sensory activity, when the senses interact directly with an object, involves also memory and imagination and does so very vividly; later they appear as only shadows and secondary products of the sensory activity proper. On the contrary, the sensory activity reaches its highest level when its product approximates direct sensory perception. I assume that the difference between the primary and the secondary activity of the sense is accounted for by the fact that during the primary activity real movements and sensations occur in the eye, whereas during secondary activity only the intended movements and sensations take place. Thus, for example, in the first case the eye follows the outlines of an object with real movements whereas in the second case only the intended movements take place without realization of the movement proper.

This kind of movement is observed more readily in the organs of speech when we surprise ourselves during soliloquy. In a less refined way one can observe this activity in larger muscle groups. For example, the muscles of the extremities tend to be stimulated for action when bases for external or internal muscular impulses are being inhibited by the will. In general one may expect that each actual movement must correspond to an intended parallel, just as every free force of nature corresponds to a constrained one, without being in principle different on this account. These concepts were formulated long ago in physics, driven by such phenomena as weight, latent temperature, electricity and magnetism, or mutually limiting tensions and tendencies. The same applies to intended sensations. Each sensation is a particular modification of the awareness of one's feeling of identity by external limitations. The tendency to bring about such a specific limitation by an inner stimulus would constitute the intended sensation.

The intended movements and sensations, like their originals, are mediated by the apparatus of movement and the sensory organs.

It is unnecessary to assign to memory and imagination and their varieties to specific organs in the brain. The subjects of both as well as the direct sensations have been specified in minute detail. Why would one wish to assign them to specific organs in the brain, the detailed structure of which is so little known? It would make the whole issue even more incomprehensible. The brain appears to be the seat and collector of the general free principle flowing into all other organs, which receives its particular specificity only in these organs.

For a long time the senses were represented as animals within an animal. They were assigned their particular individualities that, however, in addition to their own functions are controlled by a higher principle, which accounts for the unity of action and consciousness.

Where this unifying principle releases its ties, there immediately emerges subordinate activity of its own. Many a folly and madness may be viewed as the result of the separation of one or more sensory and motor organs from the unity of mental activity. In this way its products become dissociated and its activities appear to lack purpose in attacking the harmony of the rest of the organism. Even during sleep the individual senses appear to follow different paths as we readily establish when we observe ourselves as we are falling asleep: Frequently the eye and the ear dream different dreams at the same time. It is also relevant that usually the dreams deal with images mediated by the senses that were most active before sleep.

What I have just said about the senses in general applies to the eyes in particular. Throughout this book I have been concerned with what goes on in the organ of vision and, more specifically, in its physiological operation. However, I shall close by pointing to the soul of this sense and its relation to a higher principle.

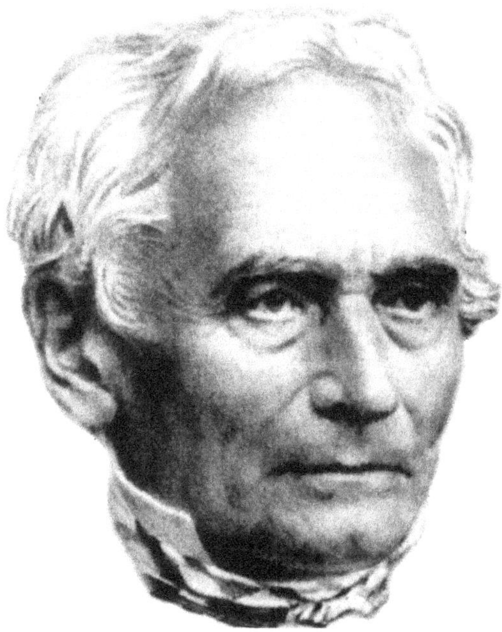

FIG. 5.1. Portrait of Purkinje in 1862, after an illustration in Hykeš (1936).

5

Assessment

The 19th century heralded exciting times for neuroscience. The experimental methods that had proved so successful in the physical and chemical sciences were applied to biology; nerve structures and pathways were charted; the functions of the brain were hinted at by Gall, who even proposed that psychological faculties were localized in specific regions of the cerebrum; and perceptual phenomena were given physiological interpretations. Purkinje participated in several of these developments, although the principal focus of this book is on the last mentioned, which was the topic of Purkinje's doctoral dissertation of 1818, which was printed in 1819 and reprinted in 1823.

The scope of Purkinje's interests was broad, and he made important contributions to many areas that have hardly been touched on. For example, in his inaugural address at Breslau, Purkinje (1823b) described the principles on which an ophthalmoscope could operate, and he outlined how fingerprints could be used as a means of identifying individuals. He found "after examining a great number of individuals, nine patterns of papillary lines on the skin of the fingers" (*Opera Selecta*, Purkinje, 1948, p. XXIV). The nine patterns are shown in Fig. 5.2.

Two years later, working without the aid of a good achromatic microscope, Purkinje (1825b) discovered the germinal vesicle in the yolk of bird's eggs.

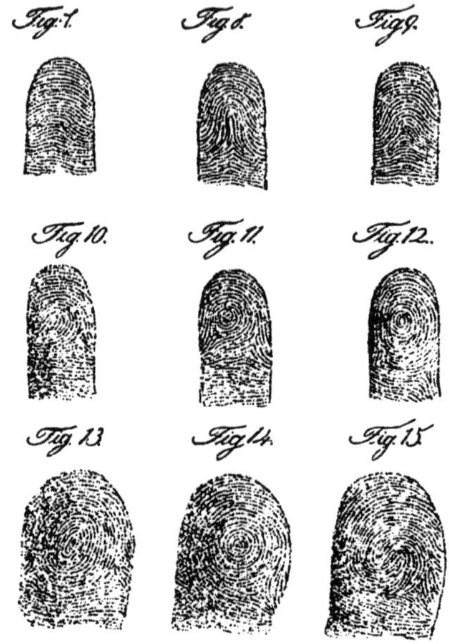

FIG. 5.2. Nine patterns of fingerprints, from Purkinje (1823b).

He also introduced the term protoplasm at around the same time. Sleep was among the topics he examined in his earliest publications and he returned to it over two decades later, when he speculated on the neural nature of sleep and wakefulness (Purkinje, 1846b); sleep resulted when the flow through the sensory systems to the cortex was inhibited. Nonetheless, Purkinje remains best known for the structures and phenomena with which his name is linked. Many of these had been observed before his time, but Purkinje's vision yielded more precise descriptions of them and laid bare their significance. That is, Purkinje saw further than his peers both literally and metaphorically. The existence of earlier descriptions should be noted with these points in mind.

Some of Purkinje's images, the reflections from the surfaces of the eye, had been described and utilized before Purkinje. In 1801 Young observed the reflections of a candle flame from the corneal surface of the eye and noted that its shape did not change with accommodation, thus excluding variations in corneal curvature from focusing on objects at different distances. In 1808 Brewster used the reflections of a candle flame to determine changes in the curvature of the cornea in a case of keratoconus (see Wardrop, 1808, 1818). However, the intensity of the reflected images decline as they pass through more media and so, as Helmholtz noted, "The surfaces of the crystalline lens also reflect some light, but not very much" (2000a, p. 19). Helmholtz made only passing reference to Purkinje's observations of the images, but Donders (1864) suitably acknowledged

Purkinje's discovery. Sanson (1838) described the use of the reflected images in the diagnosis of cataract, and they are sometimes referred to Purkinje–Sanson images. Of the four images, one is inverted (that from the posterior surface of the lens, which is concave) and one (from the posterior corneal surface) is very indistinct, because the refractive indices of the cornea and aqueous humor are very similar.

Throughout the time Purkinje was writing on vision, the mechanism of accommodation remained an issue of great debate. He used the evidence from image reflections as well as from the effects of belladonna to support Young's theory of accommodation. Belladonna was not the only narcotic the consequences of which he determined by self-administration (Votava, 1971), but it was the principal one for its effects on vision. The means by which the changes in lens curvature are controlled was elucidated later in the century by Helmholtz (1867, 2000a). To measure the curvatures of the optical surfaces in the living eye, Helmholtz invented the ophthalmometer; he confirmed the speculations of Descartes and the experiments of Young and Cramer that the lens changes curvature, and he described how this is achieved. "On contraction, the ciliary muscle could pull the posterior end of the zonule forwards nearer the lens and reduce the tension of the zonule. . . . If the pull of the zonule is relaxed in accommodating for near vision, the equatorial diameter of the lens will diminish, and the lens will get thicker in the middle, both surfaces becoming more curved" (Helmholtz, 2000a, p. 151).

The Purkinje shift had its precursors, too. Before the description by Purkinje's contemporary, Klotz, Aristotle had made a similar, though less precise, observation: "We never see a colour in absolute purity: it is always blent, if not with another colour, then with rays of light or with shadows, and so it assumes a new tint. That is why objects assume different tints when seen in light and sunshine, and according as the rays of light are strong or weak" (Ross, 1913, p. 793b). According to Klemm (1911), the change in the apparent brightnesses of red and blue threads at dusk is described in the Koran. A more deliberate description of possibly the same phenomenon was given by Leonardo da Vinci: "Green and blue are invariably accentuated in the half-shadows, yellow and red and white in the light parts" (Minnaert, 1940, p. 111). However, neither of these are as clear descriptions as that given by Klotz, a translation of which is given in chapter 1. Klotz made his discovery in the context of painted pigments. Purkinje placed the color shift in the context of individual differences in color vision and the color blindness that is experienced in the peripheral retina.

Developments in microanatomy accelerated apace in the second quarter of the 19th century. The distortions attendant on using simple microscopes were bypassed with the application of achromatic lenses, making it possible to see small structures in sharper detail. Purkinje was amongst the first to appreciate this, and he was to apply his acute vision to the structures viewed with achromatic microscopes. Hence we have Purkinje cells in the brain and Purkinje fibers around the heart.

NEUROSCIENCE

The origins of neuroscience stretch back to antiquity (see Finger, 1994, 2000), but particularly large strides were made in the 19th century (Wade, 2000d). The gross anatomy of the brain was clarified, and its microanatomy was subjected to achromatic scrutiny; the cell and neuron doctrines were advanced; function was related to structure, initially fancifully by Gall and later with surgical precision by Ferrier and others; and a wide range of cognitive dysfunctions were linked with abnormalities in brain structures.

Nineteenth-century neuroscience was built on the basic structures that were bared in the previous century. Galen's concept of the animal spirit, circulating between the nerves and the cerebral ventricles, had been all but banished from the conceptual armory of the fledgling neuroscientists. Toward the end of the 18th century, George Prochaska, who taught at the University of Prague before Purkinje, surveyed the history of the concept of the animal spirit, and heralded a new dawning: "We will term the cause latent in the pulp of the nerves, producing its effects, and not as yet ascertained, the *vis nervosa*: we will arrange its observed effects, which are the functions of the nervous system, and discover its laws; and thus we shall be able to found a true and useful doctrine, which will undoubtedly afford a new light, and more elegant character to medical art" (Prochaska, 1851, p. 380). Seven years after Prochaska's statement, in 1791, the frequently made suggestion that the nerves might transmit electricity was bolstered by Galvani's experiments (see Brazier, 1984, 1988; Piccolino, 1997). Galvani was able to demonstrate the muscular contraction of an isolated frog's leg without knowingly applying an electrical current. The era of animal electricity was born, and in the 19th century it was to mature into the principle of nerve transmission by means of action potentials.

Conceptual advances in 19th-century neuroscience were facilitated by the cell and the neuron doctrines. Their importance was clearly seen by Sherrington; he commenced *The Integrative Action of the Nervous System* with the statement: "Nowhere in physiology does the cell-theory reveal its presence more frequently in the very framework of the argument than at the present time in the study of nervous reactions" (1906, p. 1). Purkinje's (1837a) contribution was more than describing the cells that bear his name; he also speculated on the organization and functions of the nerve cells: "With reference to the importance of the ganglionic corpuscles, it could be suggested that they are probably central structures. This fact is likely because of their whole organization in three concentric circles [i.e., periphery of cell, nuclear membrane, and confines of the nucleolus] which may be related to the elementary brain and nerve fibres in the same way as centers of force are related to the conduction pathways of force, or like the ganglia to the nerves of the ganglion, or like the brain substance to the spinal cord and cranial nerves. This means that they would be collectors, generators, and distributors of the neural organ" (Clarke and O'Malley, 1968, p. 56). The neuron doctrine was more firmly established by evidence about the synapse, the term introduced by Sherrington, who proposed a mode of chemical transmission across the synaptic junctions.

Purkinje's contributions to the dawning neuroscience were not only at the molecular level of cellular structure but also at the molar level of exact subjectivism. The interpretation of perceptual phenomena in terms of their underlying physiology represented a novel departure. As was noted in chapter 1, the study of vision underwent a revolution in the 19th century: it was displaced from the natural environment and transferred to the laboratory. Wheatstone was particularly instrumental in this shift; he invented instruments that fractionated time (the kaleidophone and the electromagnetic chronoscope) and space (the stereoscope). Wheatstone's wider interests in vision were stimulated by Purkinje's books on subjective vision. Wheatstone noted the following (C.W., 1830):

> The physiology of vision has a peculiar claim on the attention of philosophers, as presenting some of those links which connect physical with mental phenomena. Metaphysicians, physiologists, natural philosophers, and artists, have equally made it an object of their study.... That the subject is of such equal interest to so many different classes of inquirers, is perhaps the cause that, as a whole, it is so imperfectly known.... To render some assistance towards forming a more complete theory of vision, we shall successively give an account of the discoveries of Purkinje, Goethe, Mile, Müller, Plateau, & c. (p. 102)

Wheatstone did, in fact, provide only an account of Purkinje's studies (see below); perhaps this was because his own experimental enquiries demanded more of his time.

Johannes Müller (1826b) also wrote a book on subjective visual phenomena, relating them where possible to their underlying physiology. In his *Elements of Physiology* he remarked that "of these phenomena... knowledge of which we are principally indebted to Purkinje" (1843, p. 1210), before describing some of Purkinje's observations. Müller's subsequent influence on the course of physiology in Germany was enormous (see Rothschuh, 1973; Cahan, 1993). In the 1840s the two most productive laboratories of physiology in Germany were those directed by Purkinje at Breslau and Müller at Berlin.

These experimental developments were made despite the fact both Purkinje and Müller were in thrall of *Naturphilosophie*. Purkinje was in the vanguard of experimental physiology at a time when it was considered as an adjunct to anatomy. As Kruta noted: "He was officially professor of physiology (and pathology) in a period of transition from the older concept of this branch of science, which mainly in Germany and Central Europe, was 'discursive' i.e., speculative and became eventually 'real' i.e. experimental science as physics and chemistry" (1969, p. 7).

To achieve this goal Purkinje argued for an independent institute of experimental physiology at Breslau. His initial proposals were made to the university authorities in 1831, and the institute was opened 8 years later. It was one of the first such institutes, and provided a model for others to follow. Moreover, Purkinje had a broad view of physiology, which was seen as providing the basis for a scientific understanding of medicine. In 1827 he wrote that "We should not distinguish sharply between pathology and physiology as has often been done so far, and is likely to be done for practical purposes also in the future. There are physiological and pathological functions. The former belong under the complex of normal vital processes, the later in the foreground only in unusual conditions, but are therefore not less orderly manifestations of one and the same principle" (Kruta, 1969, p. 42).

By emphasizing observation and experiment, Purkinje placed his science above his philosophy; his romantic physiology rarely intruded into his experimental physiology. The work he committed to print related to the experimental studies he conducted rather than the philosophy he followed. However, the distinction would not have been so sharp for him. Subjective experience and experiments based on such observations were considered as legitimate methods of physiological research, and they could yield physiological insights. Purkinje followed Gruithuisen in using the term *heautognostisch* to signify such experiments of self-exploration. Among the subjective experiences he examined early in his career were those of drugs, vertigo, and vision.

In the context of his experiments on self-administered drugs, Purkinje also sought to link normal physiology with pathology. If the operation of drugs on a healthy organism under controlled conditions of administration were known, then a more rational basis for their therapeutic application might be achieved. Before his attempts at integrating physiology with pharmacology, the latter was taught in terms of listing descriptions of the clinical effects of applying drugs. Accordingly, it was not only in the area of pathology that Purkinje's experiments broke new ground but also in that of psychopharmacology.

VERTIGO

Purkinje's experiments on vertigo have been taken as heralding a new era. A new sense, the vestibular system, was exposed by Flourens' scalpel, and Purkinje's investigations of vertigo would eventually be interpreted in the light of semicircular canal function. However, this was not achieved by Purkinje himself, despite his knowledge of Flourens' experiments. In 1826 Purkinje published a detailed review of a German translation of Flourens' (1824) book, in which Purkinje described his experiments (with his student Krauss) confirming the effects of cerebellar lesions on postural control. In the review he outlined the essential features of his earlier (1820) experiments on vertigo and sought to relate them to Flourens' experiments. At first Purkinje considered that the brain was a light substance that moved in one direction or another as a consequence of the mechanical forces acting on it. This view was changed to one in which the brain itself either had some internal disturbance or contracted, but he could find no evidence from lesions to indicate how such action took place. Lesions in the cerebellum, on the other hand, had specific effects on vertigo: "With the first repetition of Flourens' experiments on the cerebellum I was left in no doubt that the subsequent appearance of uncoordinated movements in animals was nothing other than the expression of a powerful vertigo, and that the experience of space was disturbed. The following experiments with lesions in different parts of the cerebellum similarly indicated that the direction of vertigo was so determined" (Purkinje, 1826, p. 122). In the following year Purkinje published a longer article on the physiological significance of vertigo in which these ideas were elaborated. His conclusion was that "The cerebellum has two organic functions, one works through the musculature and stimulates conscious movements, the other acts on the cerebrum and results in the combined sensation and perception of spatial experience" (1827a, p. 309). He also related these localized effects to the uncoordinated eye, head, and body movements that occur during epileptic seizures.

Similar experiments on vertigo to those that had been performed by Purkinje (1820) had been conducted decades earlier by Wells (1792, 1794a, 1794b), but were unknown both to Purkinje and to those who subsequently studied vestibular function, as was outlined in chapter 1. Indeed, in the article on vertigo of 1827 Purkinje stated that "only Darwin had investigated the true physiological significance of this phenomenon" (1827a, p. 286). Wells seems to have been destined for distinguished oblivion (see Wade, 2000c)! He suffered much the same fate with regard both to his studies on binocular visual direction and to his speculations on natural selection (see Wells, 1818). Shryock (1944) has commented on the neglect of Wells' writing in the latter domain and has examined the general reasons for the lack of scientific recognition. These included the insignificance of the authors or the power of their antagonists, the inaccessibility of the original or the obscurity of the style in which it was written, and the lack of contemporary interest that was due either to intellectual inertia or to the advanced nature of the ideas expressed.

Several of these factors could have been responsible for the neglect of Wells' experiments on vertigo. First, the title of his book describing the first series of experiments on vertigo did not advertise that fact. Its full title was *An Essay Upon Single Vision With Two Eyes: Together With Experiments and Observations on Several Other Subjects in Optics*; vertigo was one of the other subjects. The title of the particular essay was "On visible position, and visible motion"; it treated both visual orientation during changes in posture (as in sailing) and postrotary visual motion. His writing style was such that he encapsulated the essential features of vertigo in the space of a few pages. One aspect might have hindered adequate recognition of the empirical import: Afterimages were described as spectra, following Robert Darwin's (1786) usage, and this might have appeared confusing to subsequent readers of his experiments. Wells was not an insignificant figure; he was elected a Fellow of the Royal Society on the basis of his book on binocular vision. He did have a powerful antagonist in the person of Erasmus Darwin. Wells' second series of experiments on vertigo, in response to Darwin's (1794) criticisms, were reported as letters to the editor of *The Gentleman's Magazine*; it had a wide readership within Britain, and the letters were noted by Erasmus

Darwin—to whom they were directed. The magazine was unlikely to have been read farther afield, but the style in which Wells' experiments were expressed is a lesson in clarity. Which brings us to the second point: Those reading Darwin's *Zoonomia* in any of its editions or in translation would not have been presented with a balanced account of Wells' experiments. Darwin had a vested interest in supporting his and his son's theory against the empirical onslaught directed at it by Wells. Even in the context of eye movements Darwin has been accorded credit for describing postrotary nystagmus rather than Wells. Bender and Shanzer (1982) stated that "Erasmus Darwin, in his studies of vertigo, noted 'rolling movements' of both eyes, which must have been nystagmus" (p. 45). They proceeded to describe Purkinje's studies of optokinetic nystagmus, with no reference to Wells at all. The most likely reason for the neglect was that Wells' ideas were ahead of his time: There was no knowledge of the sensory system that could mediate the effects he demonstrated with such clarity. However, the same can be said of Purkinje's (1820) subjective descriptions of vertigo. Another possibility is that the early historians of the vestibular system were themselves mostly German speakers, and they relied on the material that was most readily available to them. Even Darwin's deliberations on vertigo, available in translation, were not fully absorbed into the German literature. Perhaps the most important factor was that Purkinje and Flourens were contemporaries. Purkinje's experiments were to find an interpretation in terms of the semicircular canal functions Flourens' lesions were able to uncover.

VISION

It must be rare for a published doctoral dissertation to be reviewed at length by one of the intellectual pillars of the day. Such happened to Purkinje. Goethe wrote an extensive review of it in 1824. He reprinted particular short passages from Purkinje's dissertation, and then added his own comments in parentheses. These were either of a general nature or related to Goethe's own observations. He was clearly impressed by the subtlety of Purkinje's vision because he wrote "we are grateful to the author for undertaking this task and for raising it to a new level" (1824, p. 103).

The significance of Purkinje's observations and experiments was quickly appreciated both in Germany and in other European countries. Reviews appeared in German journals following publication in 1819. They were generally positive, although a constantly repeated theme was that the observations should be confirmed by others. Goethe was not alone in his admiration of Purkinje's powers of observation. In 1826 the young experimentalist Johannes Müller extended the work in a book entitled *Über die phantastischen Gesichtserscheinungen* (*On Fantastic Visual Appearances*); in that same year he published a book on comparative physiology and eye movements (Müller, 1826a).

The latency of the response in Britain was somewhat longer, but the analysis was more detailed. Charles Wheatstone published a summary of the 1823 reprint of

Purkinje's first volume in 1830 (see Wade, 1983). Wheatstone entitled his review "Contributions to the physiology of vision," and he was to use the same title for his own classic article describing the stereoscope in 1838: "Contributions to the physiology of vision—Part the first. On some remarkable, and hitherto unobserved, phenomena of binocular vision." Wheatstone commenced his review of Purkinje's book by noting that "this little volume has excited considerable interest in Germany" (C.W., 1830, p. 102), but he took issue with the use of the term subjective:

> To distinguish these phenomena from those which arise on the presence of their appropriate external objects, the author employs the term subjective, which, as denoting this class of phenomena better than any other we are acquainted with, and, to avoid circumlocution, we have purposely retained; it will, however, on consideration, be perceived, that the term is not strictly proper, as, correctly speaking, all phenomena, *as such*, are subjective, *i.e.* in the mind; and were we, without qualification, to admit the classification of phenomena into objective and subjective, we should be unable to determine, with any degree of accuracy, where the objective ends or the subjective begins. (p. 102)

Wheatstone not only gave a summary of selected sections from Purkinje's book, but he also added novel methods for observing some phenomena—particularly the visibility of retinal blood vessels.

The title of Purkinje's doctoral dissertation was *Beiträge zur Kenntniss des Sehens in subjectiver Hinsicht* (*Contributions to the Knowledge of Vision in its Subjective Aspect*). One factor that could have influenced this title was Steinbuch's (1811) *Beytrag zur Physiologie der Sinne*, which had been studied by Purkinje and from which he drew inspiration. Why did Purkinje add a prefix to the title of the book when it was reprinted in 1823, and leave all else unchanged? The term *Beobachtungen und Versuche* was used in many earlier articles and books, some of which Purkinje had consulted. For example, the translation into German of John Elliott's book *Beobachtungen über die Sinne* (*Observations on the Senses*) was cited by Purkinje, and in the interim he had read a translation of Wells' article on the effects of belladonna on accommodation; it had the title "Beobachtungen und Versuche über das Sehen" (Wells, 1813). There is considerable overlap in the coverage of both these works by Elliot and Wells and Purkinje's observations of subjective vision. Indeed, the early work by Wells and Purkinje, particularly with regard to the investigations of vertigo, display many remarkable similarities, but history has accorded the accolades to Purkinje.

Concern with observations and experiments derived from the application of Newtonian methods to the study of natural phenomena. Indeed, one of Newton's most ardent advocates, Jean Théophile Desaguliers, summarized the situation succinctly: "All the Knowledge we have of Nature depends upon Facts; for without Observations and Experiments, our natural Philosophy would only be a Science of Terms and an unintelligible Jargon" (1745, p. v). Desaguliers applied this principal to perception as well as to physics and in so doing set in train the analysis of perceptual phenomena by the application of the methods of natural philosophy. He studied aspects of accommodation, binocular vision, and size perception (see Wade, 2000b). His approach was adopted by others and so potentially provided a platform from which experiments in the 19th century could spring. Moreover, Desaguliers was unusual in examining the perception of others besides himself: In his experiments on the influence of apparent distance on apparent size he tested naive observers. This procedure was not generally adopted until the late 19th century. Purkinje based his conclusions on the evidence of his own senses rather than on those of many.

It is evident that Purkinje's plans for a second book on subjective visual phenomena were well advanced by the time his doctoral dissertation was reprinted in 1823. As can be seen from the title page (chapter 3) he referred to it as the first small volume. Indeed, his research on accommodation and vertigo had been undertaken in the intervening years, and these are reflected in the *New Contributions*. The title page of the second volume is shown in Fig. 5.3, and its contents were listed in chapter 2. It is of interest to contrast the first and the second small volumes. The latter was more mature, with a greater appreciation of a body of existing literature

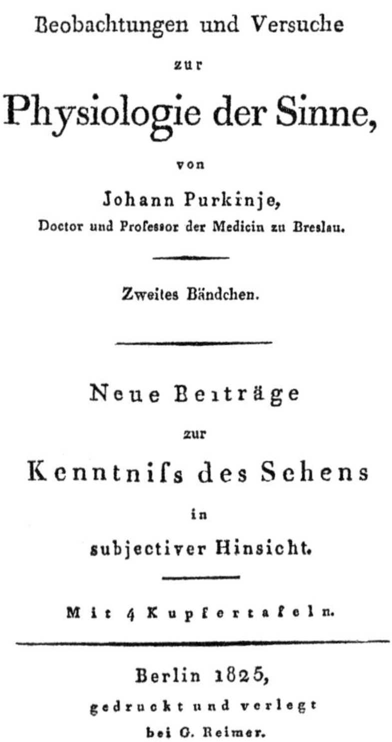
Beobachtungen und Versuche

zur

Physiologie der Sinne,

von

Johann Purkinje,

Doctor und Professor der Medicin zu Breslau.

Zweites Bändchen.

Neue Beiträge

zur

Kenntniſs des Sehens

in

subjectiver Hinsicht.

Mit 4 Kupfertafeln.

Berlin 1825,

gedruckt und verlegt

bei G. Reimer.

FIG. 5.3. Title page of Purkinje (1825a).

to which some reference was made. Many of the topics described in the first book were returned to but some were new, as was indicated in chapter 1. However, the orientation remained much the same. In the preface to the second volume Purkinje acknowledged his debt to Goethe: "If I have been lucky in making some discoveries in the domain of vision, and still have the prospect of doing more, it should be considered as the work of a journeyman following in your footsteps. Accept this true homage from one of your humblest but closest admirers."

What were the "discoveries in the domain of vision" that can be attributed to Purkinje? Those that bear his name have been discussed above, others were discussed in chapter 1, but many more are to be found in his first book on subjective vision, the text of which is translated in chapter 4. Of particular note are his observations on flicker patterns, pressure figures, effects of electrical stimulation, visibility of retinal blood vessels, afterimages, pattern distortions, and eye movements. These are dealt with in order.

Stroboscopic patterns, produced by flicker, were a novelty both in terms of their generation and their visual complexity. Purkinje called them light and shade figures, and produced them with a rotating sectored disk in addition to waving his fingers in front of the eye. He varied the characteristics of the colors and the number of sectors on the rotating disk, and found that the basic requirement was that the alternating sectors should be lighter and darker. In this regard it is strange that Purkinje did not report any color experiences because they were first described (at approximately the same time) with rotating or oscillating black and white patterns (see Wade, 1977a, 1998a). They are now called subjective colors, despite the fact that all color perception is subjective, as Newton noted. The reason that the term is still applied is because the stimulus does not have the variations in wavelength that would be expected from the colors perceived.

The history of subjective colors is a fascinating one, although it relates to the period after which Purkinje's book was written. According to Erb and Dallenbach (1939) and Cohen and Gordon (1949), the phenomenon was discovered independently many times, largely because of the wide range of stimuli that can induce the colors. They are often referred to as Fechner colors, following his description of the colors seen in a rotating black and white disk: "Rapidly rotate a disc covered with variations in black and white and one sees colors. . . . However, the impressions of the different colors disappear at different rates" (Fechner, 1838, pp. 227–228). Fechner himself was most surprised to see the colors, because he was using the disk, with different sectors of black, as a means of producing gradations of gray during rotation. Having experienced the colors, he confirmed their appearance by asking other people to look at the rotating disk; they described the colors in similar terms, although there were considerable differences in their apparent intensities. This led Fechner to realize that the phenomenon must have a lawful basis, and he studied the effect of angular velocity on the colors seen as well as variations in the number of sectors on the disk. He remarked, ruefully, that Goethe would have liked the phenomenon, as colors could be produced from black and white! As a final footnote to his paper, Fechner expressed surprise that Talbot (1834) had not noticed the phenomenon during his photometric experiments, which involved rotating similar disks to produce a gradation of grays. It is even more surprising that so astute an observer as Purkinje failed to describe the color experience. As we will note later, such subjective colors can also be experienced with the finely engraved parallel lines used by Purkinje to produce pattern distortions.

Pressure figures had been described many times previously, but they had not been examined with the scrutiny that Purkinje applied to them, nor perhaps with the pressure! It is evident from his descriptions that he must at times have produced temporary blindness, which is now known to be due to retinal anoxia. Indeed, it has been used as a means of establishing the central basis for interocular transfer of motion aftereffects (Barlow and Brindley, 1963). Interocular effects were described under several headings by Purkinje, and these occasionally refer to effects that would now be called binocular rivalry. However, the discussions of binocular vision are in the traditional mode of accounting for singleness of vision rather than stereopsis. Purkinje did use the term stereometric but it was not applied in the systematic manner in which Wheatstone (1838) was to expose and express it.

Galvanic light patterns had been described by Volta (1800) and by Ritter (1801, 1805), but not in the detail provided by Purkinje, who made extensive reference to Ritter's work when he returned to the topic in the *New Contributions* of 1825. Purkinje reported that the color effects were easier to observe when the direction of the voltaic current was interrupted by moving the electrodes around. He described the effects as similar in appearance to pressure figures, although this observation was by no means universal. Helmholtz (2000b) gave the following, somewhat jaundiced, summary: "So far as the writer is aware, these rhombs have never been seen by any other observer; and it is a question therefore whether their regular form was not due to idiosyncracies of Purkinje's eyes" (p. 18). Purkinje (1825a) also found that the effects tended to be visible around the blind spot, and he devoted 19 figures to representing his observations.

The effects of galvanic stimulation were soon to be extended by Johannes Müller (1826a, 1826b), and these studies, together with his examination of pressure figures, were instrumental in his formulation of the doctrine of specific nerve energies—that each sense organ yields its characteristic sensation regardless of how it is stimulated. Purkinje (1820) also followed Ritter in investigating the effects of electrical stimulation on vertigo, as was mentioned in chapter 1.

It is surprising that the visibility of the retinal blood vessels, the Purkinje tree, was attributed so late in the history of visual science. Pequet (1668) described the structure of the vessels in the context of Mariotte's (1668) contention that the retina was not the receptive surface for vision. Pecquet's anatomical observations were detailed, but they seem to have been shrouded by the controversy over the blind spot and not related to their observation. He wrote the following (1668):

> These Vessels, which are no other but the ramifications of the Veins and Arteries, are derived from the Heart, and having no communication with the brain, they cannot carry thither the Species of the Object. If therefore the Visual rays, issuing from an Object fall on these Vessels at the place of their Trunk or main Body, 'tis certain that the Impression made thereby will produce no Vision, and that the picture of that Object will be deficient; as when on a white paper in an obscure Chamber, there is some black spot, or in it some hole considerably bigg: for the more sensible this blackness or hole is, the more of the image of the object it intercepts from our Eyes. It is not so in respect of the *small* ramifications, that issue from those trunks and shoot into the *Retina*. For if they be met with at the place of the bottom of the Eye, where Vision is made distinct, they will not render the image of the Object deficient, because they are so small, as not to be sensible. (p. 670)

It should be noted, however, that the argument is made on logical rather than phenomenological grounds. Bell's (1803) observations were more pertinent because he appreciated that the visible ramifications were shadows on the retina cast by the vessels. Purkinje not only described them but also represented them graphically.

The visibility of shadows of retinal blood vessels cast by oblique illumination was probably confused with the occurrence of other entoptic phenomena, like flying gnats (or floaters). In fact, a diagram of what could be the Purkinje tree was published by La Hire (1694), and it is shown in Fig. 5.4. The description of the appearance, however, bore more relation to floaters than to the visibility of shadows cast by retinal blood vessels: "Presbyopes are subject to see spots and threads, like the mouches volantes that are always before the eyes, principally when looking at a white or bright object. These spots are not all of the same nature; there are those

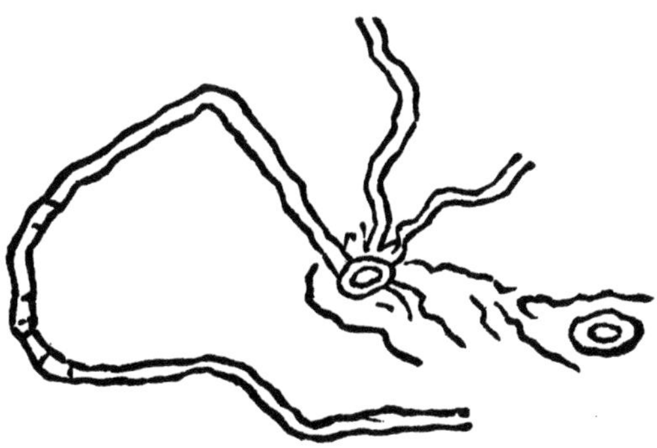

FIG. 5.4. A diagram from La Hire (1694) that could represent the large vessels of the Purkinje tree.

that I call permanent because they remain in the same position with respect to the visual axis. . . . Others float about and continually change their location" (La Hire, 1694, p. 260). The distinction between permanent and changing floaters might well indicate that the former were shadows of retinal vessels. The two concentric regions in the figure could correspond to the foveal depression (on the right of the illustration) and the optic disk (on the left).

Later in the 19th century the Purkinje tree was used by Heinrich Müller (1855) to locate the various structures in the retina and to provide evidence of the fibers connecting the receptors with the ganglion cells. Ratliff (1971), in reviewing the impact of Purkinje's approach to subjective vision in general and to this phenomenon in particular, remarked that Purkinje's observations of the retinal blood vessels "altered the character of the entire field of the study of mental phenomena" (p. 91).

Afterimages were examined in a variety of ways by Purkinje, and he devoted many pages to descriptions of their characteristics. They were given the name *Nachbild* by him, although he referred to the long-lasting effects of intense stimulation as *Blendungsbilder* (blinding images). Purkinje introduced a quantitative dimension to their study by noting the relationship between the duration of initial stimulation and that of the ensuing afterimage. He also charted the color changes that are initially visible. As the editors of his *Opera Selecta* noted: "His observations of after images was so thorough that even today the fifth phase of the after vision is called Purkyně's phase" (1948, p. XXIII). The rapid color changes that follow intense stimulation have been examined in many subsequent studies, although the terminology has not always been in accord. For example, Brown (1965) referred to the second positive phase as the Purkinje image, and it is also called Bidwell's ghost. Purkinje did make a distinction between persisting images, afterimages, and memory images, all of which he considered to be located in the retina. That the "seat of vision" was located so peripherally was a common assumption in the early 19th century because so little was known about the functions of the brain.

The pattern distortions visible during or after observation of geometrical patterns were studied by Purkinje for the first time. A variety of such distortions is now known to occur (see Wade, 1977b); the effects and the aftereffects were not only described by Purkinje but he also attempted to account for them by manipulating the conditions under which they can be seen. For example, he found that the aftereffects were dependent on the line spacing (spatial frequency) of the gratings. The perceptual transformation of parallel lines into wavy ones was accounted for by the overlap of real images with slightly displaced afterimages, like optical interference fringes. Thus afterimages assumed an interpretive as well as a phenomenological role. There has been a resurgence of interest in these phenomena as a consequence of their use by artists (see Wade, 1982) and their examination by visual scientists (Zeki, 1999). For example, the patterns of brain activity when one is observing the apparent motion visible in patterns like Fig. 5.5, particularly in the white annuli, indicate increased activity in the region (V5) associated with the detection of real movement.

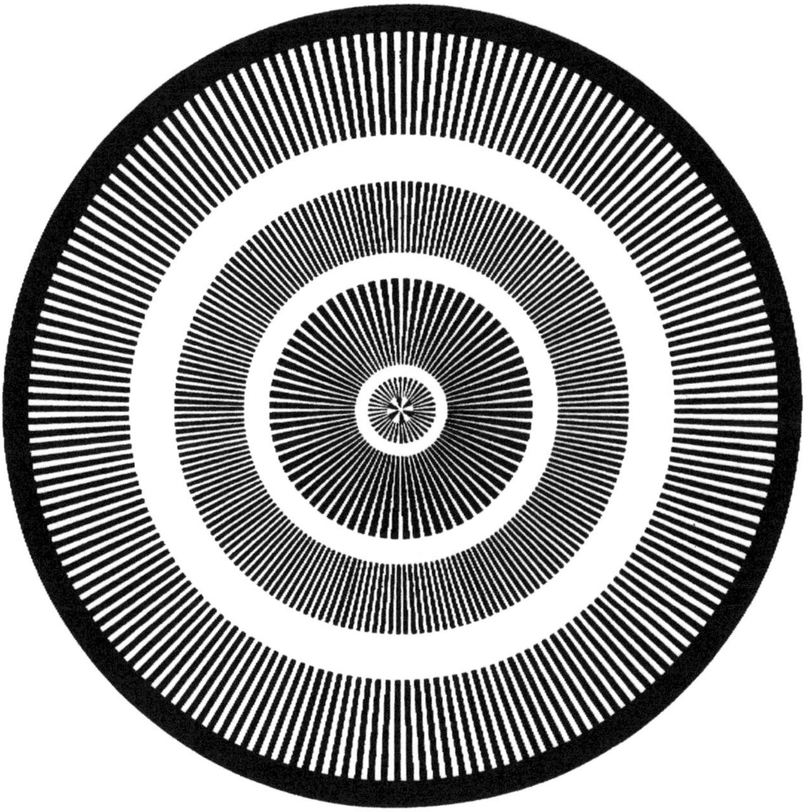

FIG. 5.5. A pattern of radiating lines in which apparent motion of scintillating dots can be seen, particularly in the white annuli.

It was noted earlier that Purkinje did not report seeing colors in rotating black and white patterns. A similar surprise is encountered when one examines his reports of pattern distortions. The parallel lines in fine engravings were precisely the stimuli used by Brewster (1825) to induce subjective colors: "When the eye is stedfastly fixed, for some time, upon the parallel lines which are generally used to represent the sea in maps, the lines will all break into serpentine lines, and *red*, *yellow*, *green*, and *blue* tints will appear in the interstices of them" (p. 292). Oscillating black and white lines also produced subjective colors, as Wheatstone described: "If a sheet of paper, with black characters, either printed or written, be moved rapidly backwards and forwards at the ordinary distance of distinct vision, the lines described by the motion will appear accompanied by very evident colours, the green and red obviously predominating. The experiment succeeds better if the lines are far apart, and perpendicular to the direction of motion" (C.W., 1831, p. 537).

Despite the ease with which another person's eye movements can be observed, Purkinje devoted most of his descriptions to the impressions he could determine from the movements of his own eyes. That is, he spurned the objective evidence from the eyes of others to concentrate on his own subjective impressions. In his discussion of eye movements Purkinje appreciated that edges, outlines, and intersections were regions of patterns to which the eyes were directed. He also drew attention to anisotropies of eye movements: Vertical lines could be followed most easily, then horizontal, then the intermediate orientations. Vertigo has a pronounced oculomotor component to it, but it was not mentioned by Purkinje in his first book. As noted in chapter 1, vertigo was examined in some detail by Purkinje (1820). However, more attention was paid to the subjective impressions of motion than to any attempts to note the pattern of eye movements that followed rotation.

Purkinje did not display a detailed knowledge of physiological optics that was available in his day. Thomas Young, writing two decades earlier, discussed some effects bearing great similarity to those of Purkinje, but Young interpreted them in optical rather than physiological terms. For example, Young (1801) determined the astigmatism in his own eye and was able to attribute a variety of appearances to this aberration. In like manner, Purkinje's extensive studies of afterimages did not lead to the insight that these could be used as stabilized retinal images, as Wells (1792) had appreciated. However, Purkinje did describe the perceptual fading that occurs as a consequence of steady fixation.

The description of subjective phenomena might seem to be both simple and straightforward and therefore not worthy of the acclaim directed to Purkinje. There is no better way to conclude otherwise than to repeat Helmholtz's assessment: "It might seem that nothing could be easier than to be conscious of one's own sensations; and yet experience shows that for the discovery of subjective sensations some special talent is needed, such as Purkinje manifested in the highest degree" (2000c, p. 6).

History has been deservedly kind to Purkinje. He did not see further than others by standing on the shoulders of giants; he looked inward and discovered a visual world that is still being explored.

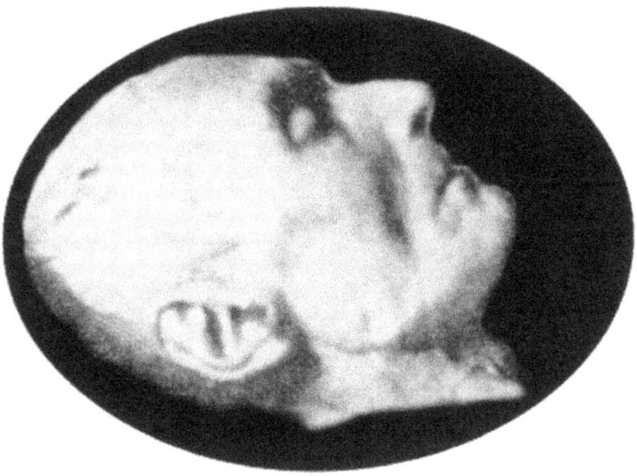

FIG. 5.6. Purkinje in repose in 1869, after a photograph in Vavroušek, Hykeš, and Noval (1937).

References

Ægineta, P. (1844). *The seven books of Paulus Ægineta*, (Vol. 1. F. Adams, Trans.). London: The Sydenham Society.

Aguilonius, F. (1613). *Opticorum libri sex. Philosophis juxta ac mathematicis utiles.* Antwerp, Belgium: Moreti.

Anon. (1972). Purkinje-Phänomen. *Brockhaus Enzyklopädie* (Vol. 15, 17th ed.). (p. 269). Wiesbaden, Germany: Brockhaus.

Ariotti, P. E. (1973). A little known early seventeenth century treatise on vision: Benedetto Castelli's Discorso sopra la Vista. *Annals of Science*, *30*, 1–30.

Aubert, H. (1888). *Physiologische Studien über die Orientierung*. Tübingen, Germany: Laupp.

Bacon, F. (1627). *Sylva sylvarum: Or a naturall historie*. London: Lee.

Bárány, R. (1913). Der Schwindel und seine Beziehungen zum Bogengangapparat des inneren Ohres. *Naturwissenschaften*, *1*, 369–401.

Barlow, H. B., & Brindley, G. S. (1963). Interocular transfer of movement aftereffects during pressure blinding of the stimulated eye. *Nature* (*London*), *200*, 1347.

Bartisch, G. (1583). *ΟΦΘΑΛΜΟΔΟΥΛΕΙΑ Das ist, Augendienst*. Dresden: Stockel.

Bell, C. (1803). *The anatomy of the human body* (Vol. 3). London: Longman, Rees, Cadell and Davies.

Bell, C. (1823). On the motions of the eye, in illustration of the uses of the muscles and of the orbit. *Philosophical Transactions of the Royal Society*, *113*, 166–186.

Bender, M. B., & Shanzer, S. (1982). History of binocular movements. In F. C. Rose & W. F. Bynum (Eds.), *Historical aspects of the neurosciences. A Festschrift for Macdonald Critchley* (pp. 45–54). New York: Raven.

Boerhaave, H. (1703). *Oratio de usu ratiocinii mechani in medicina*. Leiden: Teering.

Boring, E. G. (1942). *Sensation and perception in the history of experimental psychology*. New York: Appleton-Century.

Brazier, M. A. B. (1984). *A history of neurophysiology in the 17th and 18th centuries: From concept to experiment*. New York: Raven.

Brazier, M. A. B. (1988). *A history of neurophysiology in the 19th century*. New York: Raven.

Breuer, J. (1874). Über die Funktion der Bogengänge des Ohrlabyrinthes. *Wiener medizinisches Jahrbuch, 4*, 72–124.

Brewster, D. (1818). On a singular affection of the eye in the healthy state, in consequence of which it loses the power of seeing objects within the sphere of distinct vision. *Annals of Philosophy, 11*,151.

Brewster, D. (1825). On some remarkable affections of the retina, as exhibited in its insensibility to indirect impressions, and to the impressions of attenuated light. *Edinburgh Journal of Science, 3*, 288–293.

Brown, A. Crum (1874). Preliminary note on the sense of rotation and the function of the semicircular canals of the internal ear. *Proceedings of the Royal Society of Edinburgh, 8*, 255–257.

Brown, A. Crum (1875). On the sense of rotation and the anatomy and physiology of the semicircular canals of the internal ear. *Journal of Anatomy and Physiology, 8*, 327–331.

Brown, J. L. (1965). Afterimages. In C. H. Graham, N. R. Bartlett, J. L. Brown, Y. Hsia, C. G. Mueller, & L. A. Riggs (Eds.), *Vision and visual perception* (pp. 479–503). New York: Wiley.

Brožek, J. (1971). Purkyně and psychology in a historical research perspective. In V. Kruta (Ed.), *Jan Evangelista Purkyně 1787–1869. Centenary symposium* (pp. 105–118). Brno, Czechoslovakia: Universita Jana Evangelisty Purkyně.

Brožek, J. (1973). Whatever happened to the physiological psychology of J. E. Purkinje? In J. Linhart (Ed.), *Proceedings of the 2nd Prague Conference, Psychology of Human Learning and Problem Solving* (pp. 481–483). Prague: Charles University and the Psychological Institute of the Czechoslovak Academy of Sciences.

Brožek, J. (1988). A contribution by J. E. Purkinje (1787–1869) to the history of psychology. *History of Psychology Newsletter, 20* (1–2), 32–36.

Brožek, J. (1989). Contributions to the history of psychology: LII. Purkinje phenomenon: The original and a later account. *Perceptual and Motor Skills, 68*, 566.

Brožek, J. (1989). Psychologie, objektive. In J. Ritter and K. Gruender (Eds.), *Historisches Woerterbuch der Philosophie*. Basel, Switzerland: Schwabe.

Brožek, J. (1990). Early uses of the term "objective psychology." *Perceptual and Motor Skills, 70*, 377–378.

Brožek, J., & Hoskovec, J. (1987). *J. E. Purkyně and psychology*. Prague: Academia.

Brožek, J., & Hoskovec, J. (1988, in Czech). Purkinje's manuscripts on psychology: Content and significance. History of Science and Technology, Prague, *21* (3), 129–135.

Brožek, J., & Kuthan, V. (1990). Contributions to the history of psychology: LXXI. "Purkinje phenomenon": The genesis and the early uses of the term in French, German, and English. *Perceptual and Motor Skills, 71*, 1253–1254.

Brožek, J., Kuthan V., & Arens, K. (1991). Contributions to the history of psychology: LXXXIII. J. E. Purkinje and Mathias Klotz: Who first described "the phenomenon"? *Perceptual and Motor Skills, 73*, 511–514.

Buffon, Comte de (1743). Dissertation sur les couleurs accidentelles. *Mémoires de Mathématique et de Physique de l'Académie Royale des Sciences*, 147–158.

Burdach, K. F. (1819). *Vom Baue und Leben des Gehirns*. (Vol. 1). Leipzig: Dyk'schen Buchhandlung.

Burdach, K. F. (1822). *Vom Baue und Leben des Gehirns*. (Vol. 2). Leipzig: Dyk'schen Buchhandlung.

Burdach, K. F. (1826). *Vom Baue und Leben des Gehirns*. (Vol. 3). Leipzig: Dyk'schen Buchhandlung.

Burke, R. B. (1928). *The Opus Majus of Roger Bacon*. Philadelphia: University of Pennsylvania Press.

Burton, H. E. (1945). The Optics of Euclid. *Journal of the Optical Society of America, 35*, 357–372.

Cahan, D. (Ed.). (1993). *Hermann von Helmholtz and the foundations of nineteenth-century science*. Berkeley, CA: University of California Press.

Clarke, E., & O'Malley, C. D. (1968). *The human brain and spinal cord*. Berkeley, CA: University of California Press.

Cohen, B. (1984). Erasmus Darwin's observations on rotation and vertigo. *Human Neurobiology, 3,* 121–128.
Cohen, J., & Gordon, D. A. (1949). The Prevost–Fechner–Benham subjective colors. *Psychological Bulletin, 46,* 97–133.
Cox, J. M. (1804). *Practical observations on insanity.* London: Baldwin and Murray.
Crombie, A. C. (1967). The mechanistic hypothesis and the scientific study of vision: Some optical ideas as a background to the invention of the microscope. In S. Bradbury & G. L'E. Turner (Eds.), *Historical aspects of microscopy* (pp. 3–112). Cambridge, England: Heffer.
C.W. (1830). Contributions to the physiology of vision. No I. *Journal of the Royal Institution of Great Britain, 1,* 101–117.
C. W. (1831). Contributions to the physiology of vision. No II. *Journal of the Royal Institution of Great Britain, 1,* 534–537.
D'Arcy, Chevalier. (1765). Mémoire sur la durée de la sensation de la vue. *Mémoire de l'Académie des Science de Paris,* 439–451.
Darwin, E. (1794). *Zoonomia; or, the laws of organic life* (Vol 1). London: Johnson.
Darwin, E. (1795). *Zoonomia, oder, Gesetze des organischen Lebens.* (J. D. von Brandis, Trans.). Hannover: Hahn.
Darwin, E. (1796). *Zoonomia; or, the laws of organic life* (Vol. 1, 2nd ed.). London: Johnson.
Darwin, E. (1801a). *Zoonomia; or, the laws of organic life* (Vol. 1, 3rd ed.). London: Johnson.
Darwin, E. (1801b). *Zoonomia; or, the laws of organic life* (Vol. 4, 3rd ed.). London: Johnson.
Darwin, R. W. (1786). New experiments on the ocular spectra of light and colours. *Philosophical Transactions of the Royal Society, 76,* 313–348.
Desaguliers, J. T. (1716). A plain and easy experiment to confirm Sir Isaac Newton's doctrine of the different refrangibility of the rays of light. *Philosophical Transactions of the Royal Society, 34,* 448–452
Desaguliers, J. T. (1719). *Lectures of experimental philosophy.* London: Mears, Creake, and Sackfield.
Desaguliers, J. T. (1745). *A course of experimental philosophy* (Vol. 1, 2nd ed.). London: Innys, Longman, Shewell, Hitch, and Senex.
Descartes, R. (1637/1902). La dioptrique. In C. Adam & P. Tannery (Eds.), *Oeuvres de Descartes* (Vol. 6, pp. 81–228). Paris: Cerf.
Descartes, R. (1662). *De homine figuris et latinitate.* (F. Schuyl, Trans.). Leiden: Leffen & Moyardum.
Descartes, R. (1664/1909). Traité de l'homme. In C. Adam & P. Tannery (Eds.), *Oeuvres de Descartes* (Vol. 11, pp. 119–215). Paris: Cerf.
Dewhurst, K. (1980). *Thomas Willis's Oxford lectures.* Oxford, England: Sandford.
Diogenes Laertius (1925). *Lives of eminent philosophers* (R. D. Hicks, Trans.). London: Heinemann.
Donders, F. C. (1864). *On the anomalies of accommodation and refraction of the eye* (W. D. Moore, Trans.). Boston: Milford House.
Dostalek, K. C. (1972, in Czech). Toward the history of conditioned reflexes, *Ceskoslovenska Psychologie, 16*(3), 193–201.
Dostalek, C. (1976, in Czech). Temporary and intensity relations of the stimuli during the formation of conditioned responses. *Studies of the Czechoslovak Academy of Sciences,* No. 8. Prague: Academia.
Duke–Elder, S., & Wybar, K. (1973). *System of ophthalmology. Volume 6. Ocular motility and strabismus.* London: Kimpton.
Dusser de Barenne, J. G. (1934). The labyrinthine and postural mechanisms. In C. Murchison (Ed.) *A handbook of general experimental psychology* (pp. 204–246). New York: Russell & Russell.
Du Tour, E.-F. (1760). Discussion d'une question d'optique. *Académie des Sciences. Mémoires de Mathématique et de Physique Présentés pars Divers Savants, 3,* 514–530.
Du Tour, E.-F. (1761). Addition au Mémoire intitulé. Discussion d'une question d'optique. *Académie des Sciences. Mémoires de Mathématique et de Physique Présentés pars Divers Savants, 4,* 499–511.
Eichel, J. (1774). *Experimenta circa sensum videndi.* Collectanea Societatis Medicae Havniensis.

Elliott, J. (1780). *Philosophical observations on the senses of vision and hearing*. London: Murray.
Elliott, J. (1785). *Beobachtungen über die Sinne*. Leipzig: Weygand.
Emmert, E. (1881). Grössenverhältnisse der Nachbilder. *Klinische Merkblatt der Augenheilkunde, 19*, 443–450.
Erb, M. B., & Dallenbach, K. M. (1939). "Subjective" colors from line patterns. *American Journal of Psychology, 52*, 227–241.
Fancher, R. E. (1990). *Pioneers of psychology* (2nd ed.). New York: Norton.
Fechner, G. T. (1838). Ueber eine Scheibe zur Erzeugung subjectiver Farben. *Annalen der Physik und Chemie, 45*, 227–232.
Fechner, G.T. (1840). Ueber die subjectiven Nachbilder und Nebenbilder. *Annalen der Physik und Chemie, 50*, 193–221.
Fichte, J. G. (1794). *Einige Vorlesungen über die Bestimmung des Gelehrten*. Jena: Gabler.
Fichte, J. G. (1800). *Über die Bestimmung des Menschen zur unbeschränkten seelischen Freiheit*. Berlin: Voss.
Finger, S. (1994). *Origins of neuroscience. A history of explorations into brain function*. New York: Oxford University Press.
Finger, S. (2000). *Minds behind the brain. A history of the pioneers and their discoveries*. Oxford, England: Oxford University Press.
Flourens, M. J. P. (1824). *Recherches expérimentales sur les propriétés et les fonctions du système nerveux dans les animaux vertébrés*. Paris: Baillière.
Flourens, M. J. P. (1830). Expériences sur les canaux semi-circulaires de l'orielle. *Mémoires de l'Académie Royale des Sciences, 9*, 455.
Flourens, M. J. P. (1842). *Recherches expérimentales sur les propriétés et les fonctions du système nerveux dans les animaux vertébrés* (2nd ed.). Paris: Baillière.
Franklin, B. (1765/1970). Letter to Lord Kames. In A. H. Smyth, (Ed.), *The writings of Benjamin Franklin. Volume IX. 1783–1788*. New York: Haskell House.
Franklin, B. (1785/1970). Letter to George Whatley. In A. H. Smyth, (Ed.). *The writings of Benjamin Franklin. Volume IV. 1760–1766*. New York: Haskell House.
Franz, S. I. (1899). After-images. *Psychological Review. Monograph Supplements 3*, 1–61.
Gall, F. J. (1825). *Sur les fonctions du cerveau et sur chacune de ses parties*. Paris: Baillière.
Gall, F. J., & Spurzheim, J. C. (1810). *Anatomie et physiologie du systême nerveux en general, et du cerveau en particulier* (Vol. 1). Paris: Schoell.
Goethe, J. W. (1810). *Zur Farbenlehre*. Tübingen, Germany: Cotta.
Goethe, J. (1824). Das Sehen in subjectiven Hinsicht, von Purkinje, 1819. *Zur Naturwissenschaft überhaupt, besonders zur Morphologie* (pp. 102–177). Stuttgart: Cotta.
Goethe, J. W. (1840). *Theory of colours* (C. L. Eastlake, Trans.) London: Murray.
Griffith, C. R. (1922). *An historical survey of vestibular equilibration*. Urbana; IL: University of Illinois Press.
Grüsser, O.-J. (1984). J. E. Purkyně's contributions to the physiology of the visual, the vestibular and the oculomotor systems. *Human Neurobiology, 3*, 129–144.
Grüsser, O.-J., & Hagner, M. (1990). On the history of deformation phosphenes and the idea of internal light generated in the eye for the purpose of vision. *Documenta Ophthalmologica, 74*, 57–85.
Hallaran, W. S. (1818). *Practical observations on the causes and cure of insanity*. Cork: Edwards & Savage.
Harris, J. (1775). *A treatise of optics: Containing elements of the science; in two books*. London: White.
Hartley, D. (1749). *Observations on man, his frame, his duty, and his expectations*. London: Richardson.
Hatfield, G. (1990). *The natural and the normative. Theories of spatial perception from Kant to Helmholtz*. Cambridge, MA: MIT Press.
Helmholtz, H. (1867). Handbuch der physiologischen Optik. In G. Karsten, (Ed.). *Allgemeine Encyklopädie der Physik* (Vol. 9). Leipzig: Voss.

Helmholtz, H. (1873). *Popular lectures on scientific subjects* (E. Atkinson, Trans.). London: Longmans, Green.
Helmholtz, H. (1898). *Popular lectures on scientific subjects* (E. Atkinson, Trans.). (New ed.). London: Longmans, Green.
Helmholtz, H. (2000a). *Helmholtz's treatise on physiological optics* (Vol. 1). (J. P. C. Southall, Trans.). Bristol, England: Thoemmes.
Helmholtz, H. (2000b). *Helmholtz's treatise on physiological optics* (Vol. 2). (J. P. C. Southall, Trans.). Bristol, England: Thoemmes.
Helmholtz, H. (2000c). *Helmholtz's treatise on physiological optics* (Vol. 3). (J. P. C. Southall, Trans.). Bristol, England: Thoemmes.
Henn, V. (1984). E. Mach on the analysis of motion sensation. *Human Neurobiology, 3*, 145–148.
Hering, E. (1874). *Zur Lehre vom Lichtsinne*. Vienna: Gerold.
Herrnstein, R. J., & Boring, E. G. (1965). *A source book in the history of psychology*. Cambridge, MA.: Harvard University Press.
Herz, M. (1786). *Versuch über den Schwindel*. Berlin: Voss.
Hill, E. (1915). History of eyeglasses and spectacles. In C. A. Wood (Ed.) *The American Encyclopedia and Dictionary of Ophthalmology*. (Vol. 7) (pp. 4894–4953). Chicago: Cleveland Press.
Hirschberg, J. (1899). Geschichte der Augenheilkunde. In Graefe–Saemisch *Handbuch der gesamten Augenheilkunde*. (Vol. 12). Leipzig: Engelmann.
Hooke, R. (1665). *Micrographia: or some physiological descriptions of minute bodies made by magnifying glasses with observations and inquiries thereupon*. London: Martyn and Allestry.
Howard, I. P., & Rogers, B. (1995). *Binocular vision and stereopsis*. New York: Oxford University Press.
Howard, I. P., & Templeton, W. B. (1966). *Human spatial orientation*. London: Wiley.
Howard, I. P., & Wade, N. J. (1996). Ptolemy's contributions to the geometry of binocular vision. *Perception, 25*, 1189–1202.
Hykeš, O. V. (1936). Jan Evangelista Purkyně [Purkinje] [1787–1869]. *Osiris, 2*, 463–471.
Ilg, J. G. (1811). *Grundlinien der Zergliederungskunde des menschlichen Körpers*. Prague: Widtmann.
John, H. J. (1959). *Jan Evangelista Purkyně. Czech scientist and patriot 1787–1869*. Philadelphia, PA: American Philosophical Society.
Judd, D. B. (1927). A quantitative investigation of the Purkinje after-image. *American Journal of Psychology, 38*, 507–533.
Jurin, J. (1738). An essay on distinct and indistinct vision. In R. Smith, *A compleat system of opticks in four books* (pp. 115–171). Cambridge, England: published by the author.
Kant, I. (1781). *Critik der reinen Vernunft*. Riga, Hartknoch.
Kant, I. (1786). *Metaphysische Anfangsgründe der Naturwissenschaft*. Riga, Hartknoch.
Kepler, J. (1604). *Ad Vitellionem paralipomena*. Frankfurt: Marinium and Aubrii.
Kepler, J. (1611). *Dioptrice*. Augsburg: Franci.
King-Hele, D. (1977). *Doctor of revolution. The life and genius of Erasmus Darwin*. London: Faber & Faber.
King-Hele, D. (1999). *Erasmus Darwin: A life of unequalled achievement*. London: De La Mer.
Klemm, O. (1911). *Geschichte der Psychologie*. Leipzig: Teubner.
Klotz, M. (1806). *Meldung einer Farbenlehre und eines Farben-Systems*. Munich: Scherer.
Klotz, M. (1816). *Gründliche Farbenlehre*. Munich: Lindauer'schen Buchhandlung.
Koelbing, H. M. (1967). *Renaissance der Augenheilkunde. 1540–1630*. Bern: Huber.
Kornhuber, H. H. (1974). Introduction. In H. H. Kornhuber (Ed.), *Handbook of sensory physiology. Volume VI/1. Vestibular system Part 1: Basic mechanisms* (pp. 3–14). New York: Springer.
Kotek, V. & Niklicek, L. (1987). *Jan Evangelista Purkinje and his place in the history of medicine and natural sciences of the 19th century*. Prague: Academia.
Kruta, V. (1964a). *M.-J.-P. Flourens, J.-E. Purkyně et les débuts de la physiologie de la posture et de l'équilibre*. Paris: Alençonnaise.

Kruta, V. (1964b, in Czech). *Beginnings of the scientific career of J. E. Purkyně*. Brno, Czechoslovakia: Universita Jana Evangelisty Purkyně.

Kruta, V. (1966, in Czech). Goethe's and Purkinje's studies of vision. *News of the Czechoslovak Society for the History of Science and Technology, 3*, 30–35.

Kruta, V. (1969). *J. E. Purkyně [1787–1869] physiologist. A short account of his contributions to the progress of physiology with a bibliography of his works*. Prague: Czechoslovak Academy of Sciences.

Kruta, V. (Ed.) (1971). *Jan Evangelista Purkyně 1787–1869. Centenary symposium*. Brno, Czechoslovakia: Universita Jana Evangelisty Purkyně.

La Hire, P. de. (1685a). Dissertation sur la conformation de l'oeil. *Journal des Sçavans, 13*, 335–363.

La Hire, P. de. (1685b). Dissertation sur la conformation de l'oeil. *Journal des Sçavans, 13*, 398–405.

La Hire, P. de. (1694). Dissertation sur les differens accidens de la vue. In *Mémoires de Mathématique et de Physique* (pp. 233–302). Paris: Anisson.

Le Clerc, S. (1712). *Système de la vision*. Paris: Delaulne.

Leeuwenhoek, A. van. (1674). More observations from Mr. Leewenhook. *Philosophical Transactions of the Royal Society, 9*, 178–182.

Leeuwenhoek, A. van. (1675). Microscopical observations from Mr. Leewenhoeck, concerning the optick nerve. *Philosophical Transactions of the Royal Society, 9*, 378–380.

Liddell, E. G. T. (1960). *The discovery of reflexes*. Oxford, England: Clarendon.

Locke, J. (1690). *An essay concerning humane understanding*. London: Basset.

MacCurdy, E. (1938). *The notebooks of Leonardo da Vinci*. (Vol. 1). London: Cape.

Mach, E. (1873). Physiologische Versuche über den Gleichgewichtssinn des Menschen. *Sitzungsberichte der Wiener Akademie der Wissenschaften, 68*, 124–140.

Mach, E. (1875). *Grundlinien der Lehre von den Bewegungsempfindungen*. Leipzig: Engelmann.

Mariotte, E. (1668). A new discovery touching vision. *Philosophical Transactions of the Royal Society, 3*, 668–669.

Mariotte, E. (1683). An account of two letters of Mr. Perrault and Mr. Mariotte, concerning vision. *Philosophical Transactions of the Royal Society, 13*, 266–267.

Mather, G., Verstraten, F., & Anstis, S. (Eds.) (1998). *The motion after-effect: A modern perspective*. Cambridge, MA: MIT Press.

Matousek, O. (1961). J. E. Purkyněs Leben und Tätigkeit im Lichte der Berliner und Prager Archive. *Nova Acta Leopoldina, 24*,109–129.

Maurolico, F. (1611). *Photismi de lumine et umbrae*. Naples: Longi.

May, M. T. (1968). *Galen. On the usefulness of the parts of the body*. Ithaca, New York: Cornell University Press.

McHenry, L. C. (1969). *Garrison's history of neurology*. Springfield, IL: Thomas.

McKendrick, J. G., & Gray, A. A. (1900). The ear. In E. A. Schäfer (Ed.), *Textbook of physiology* (Vol. 2, pp. 1149–1205). Edinburgh: Pentland.

Minnaert M, (1940). *Light and colour in the open air* (H. M. Kremer-Priest, Trans.). London: Bell.

Morgagni, J. B. (1719). *Adversaria anatomica omnia*. Padua, Italy: Cominus.

Müller, H. (1855). Über die entoptische Wahrnehmung der Netzhautfässe, insbesonder als Beweismittel für die Lichtperception durch die nach hintern gelegenen Netzhautelemente. *Verhandlungen der physikalische-medicinische Gesellschaft zu Würzburg, 5*, 411–447.

Müller, J. (1826a). *Zur vergleichenden Physiologie des Gesichtssinnes des Menschen und der Thiere, nebst einen Versuch über die Bewegung der Augen und über den menschlichen Blick*. Leipzig: Cnobloch.

Müller, J. (1826b). *Über die phantastischen Gesichtserscheinungen*. Coblenz, Germany: Hölscher.

Müller, J. (1840). *Elements of physiology* (Vol. 1). (W. Baly, Trans.). London: Taylor and Walton.

Müller, J. (1843). *Elements of physiology* (Vol. 2). (W. Baly, Trans.). London: Taylor and Walton.

Needham, J., & Gwei-Djen, L. (1967). The optick artists of Chiangsu. In S. Bradbury & G. L'E. Turner (Eds.) *Historical aspects of microscopy*. (pp. 113–138). Cambridge, England: Heffer.

Newton, I. (1691/1829). Letter to John Locke. In Lord King, *The life of John Locke, with extracts from his correspondence, journals and common-place books*. London: Henry Colburn.

Newton, I. (1704). *Opticks: or, a treatise of the reflections, refractions, inflections and colours of light*. London: Smith and Walford.

Newton, I. (1717). *Opticks: or, a treatise of the reflections, refractions, inflections and colours of light* (2nd ed.). London: Innys.

Ono, H. (1981). On Wells' 1792 law of visual direction. *Perception and Psychophysics, 30*, 403–406.

Paré, A. (1564). *Dix livres de la chirurgie*. Paris: Le Royer.

Park, D. (1997). *The fire within the eye*. Princeton, NJ: Princeton University Press.

Pecquet, A. (1668). Answer to Mr. Mariotte. *Philosophical Transactions of the Royal Society, 3*, 669–671.

Piccolino, M. (1997). Luigi Galvani and animal electricity: two centuries after the foundation of electrophysiology. *Trends in Neurosciences, 20*, 443–448.

Piccolino, M. (2000). The bicentennial of the Voltaic battery (1800–2000): the artificial electric organ. *Trends in Neurosciences, 23*, 147–151.

Plateau, J. (1833). Des illusions sur lesquelles se fonde le petit appareil appelé récemment Phénakisticope. *Annales de Chimie et de Physique de Paris, 53*, 304–308.

Platter, F. (1583). *De corporis humani structura et usu*. Basel, Switzerland: König.

Pliny. (1940). *Natural history* (Vol. 3, Books VIII–XI). (H. Rackham, Trans.). London: Heinemann.

Porta, J. B. (1593). *De refractione. Optices parte. Libri novem*. Naples: Carlinum and Pacem.

Porterfield, W. (1737). An essay concerning the motions of our eyes. Part I. Of their external motions. *Edinburgh Medical Essays and Observations, 3*, 160–263.

Porterfield, W. (1738). An essay concerning the motions of our eyes. Part II. Of their internal motions. *Edinburgh Medical Essays and Observations, 4*, 124–294.

Porterfield, W. (1759). *A treatise on the eye, the manner and phænomena of vision*. Edinburgh: Hamilton and Balfour.

Priestley, J. (1772). *The history and present state of discoveries relating to vision, light, and colours*. London: Johnson.

Priestley, J. (1776). *Geschichte der Optik*. (G. S. Klügel, Trans.). Leipzig: Junius.

Prochaska, G. (1851). *A dissertation on the functions of the nervous system*. (T. Laycock, Trans). (pp. 361–450). London: The Sydenham Society.

Psotníčková, J. (1955, in Czech). *Jan Evangelista Purkyně*. Prague: Orbis.

Purkinje, J. (1819). *Beiträge zur Kenntniss des Sehens in subjectiver Hinsicht*. Prague: Vetterl.

Purkinje, J. (1820). Beyträge zur näheren Kenntniss des Schwindels aus heautognostischen Daten. *Medicinische Jahrbücher des kaiserlich-königlichen öesterreichischen Staates, 6*, 79–125.

Purkinje, J. (1823a). *Beobachtungen und Versuche zur Physiologie der Sinne. Beiträge zur Kenntniss des Sehens in subjectiver Hinsicht*. Prague: Calve.

Purkinje, J. (1823b). *De examine physiologico organi visus et systematis cutanei*. Breslau: University of Breslau.

Purkinje, J. (1825a). *Beobachtungen und Versuche zur Physiologie der Sinne. Neue Beiträge zur Kenntniss des Sehens in subjectiver Hinsicht*. Berlin: Reimer.

Purkinje, J. (1825b). *Symbolae ad ovi avium historum ante incubationem*. Breslau: University of Breslau.

Purkinje, J. (1826). Flourens de physiologia systemis nervorum. *Kritisches Repertorium für die gesammte Heilkunde, 11*, 101–123.

Purkinje, J. (1827a). Ueber die physiologische Bedeutung des Schwindels und die Beziehung desselben zu den neuesten Versuchen über die Hirnfunctionen. *Magazin für die gesammte Heilkunde, 23*, 284–310.

Purkinje, J. E. (1827b). Review of Johannes Müller's, Zur Vergleichenden Physiologie des Gesichtsinnes, 1826, und Ueber die phantastischen Gesichtserscheinungen, 1826. *Jahrbuecher fuer wissenschaftliche Kritik, 1*, 190–228.

Purkinje, J. E. (1828a). Review of C. T. Tourtual's Die Sinne des Menschen, *Jahrbuecher fuer wissenschafliche Kritik, 2*, 641–649.

Purkinje, J. E. (1828b). Ueber die Verdienste Berkeley's und die Theorie des Sehens. *Uebersicht der Arbeiten der Schlesischen Gesellschaft fuer vaterlaendische Kultur* (p. 50). Breslau.

Purkinje, J. (1830). *Symbolae ad ovi avium historum ante incubationem.* (2nd ed.). Leipzig: Voss.

Purkinje, J. (1833). Review of Burdach's Die Physiologie der Erfahrungswissenschaft. *Jahrbuecher für wissenschafliche Kritik, 1*, 789–796.

Purkinje, J. (1837a). Anatomisch-physiologische Verhandlungen. *Bericht über die Versammlung deutscher Naturforscher und Ärtze*, pp. 177–180.

Purkinje, J. E. (1837b). Review of C. G. Ehrenberg's Beobachtung einer auffallenden bisher unbekannten Structur des Seelenorgans beim Menschen. *Jahrbuecher fuer wissenschaftliche Kritik, I*, 149–160.

Purkinje, J. E. (1837c, in Czech). On the ideal nature of visual space. *Casopis ceskeho museum, 11*, 191–201.

Purkinje, J. E. (1840, in Czech). Further psychological investigations on visual space. *Casopis ceskeho museum, 14*, 355–375.

Purkinje, J. E. (1846a). Sinne in allgemeinen. In R. Wagner (Ed.), *Handwörterbuch der Physiologie.* (Vol. 3, pp. 352–359). Braunschweig, Germany: Vieweg.

Purkinje, J. (1846b). Wachen, Schlaf, Traum und verwandte Zustände. In R. Wagner (Ed.), *Handwörterbuch der Physiologie* (vol. 3, pp. 412–480). Braunschweig, Germany: Vieweg.

Purkinje, J. E. (1851, in Czech). The concept of physiology. *Casopis ceskeho museum, 25*(1), 94–112.

Purkinje, J. E. (1852). Ueber den Begriff der Physiologie. *Vierteljahrschrift fuer die praktische Heilkunde, Medizinische Fakultaet* (pp. 1–19). Prague.

Purkinje, J. E. (1853a, in Czech). Topology of the senses in general. *Ziva*, 193–196.

Purkinje, J. E. (1853b, in Czech). Topology of the senses in general. *Ziva*, 361–365.

Purkinje, J. E. (1854). Die Topologie der Sinne in allgemeinen. *Vierteljahrschrift fuer praktische Heilkunde, Medizinische Fakultaet* (pp. 11–16). Prague

Purkinje, J. E. (1857a, in Czech). On wakefulness, its degrees and the passage into sleep. *Casopis museum kralovstvi ceskeho, 31*, 3–22.

Purkinje, J. E. (1857b, in Czech). On the phenomena of human and animal sleep. *Casopis museum kralovstvi ceskeho, 31*, 188–200.

Purkinje, J. E. (1857c, in Czech). Physiology of sleep. *Casopis museum kralovstvi ceskeho, 31*, 333–341, 451–463.

Purkinje, J. E. (1857d, in Czech). Detailed informations of my older and newer literary, especially naturalistic works. *Ziva, 5*, 147–157, 203–213.

Purkinje, J. E. (1858, in Czech). Detailed information on my earlier and newer publications. *Ziva, 6*, 36–45, 103–109, 173–189, 242–246.

Purkinje, J. E. (1860). Ueber die Verwertung der bisherigen Beobachtungen im Gebiet des subjektiven Sehens. *Berichte der Koeniglichen Boehmischen Gesellschaft fuer Wissenschaften, Naturwissenschaft, mathematische Section*, Oct., 34–37.

Purkinje, J. E. (1864, in Czech). Man's individual mental mechanism. *Krok, 1*, 7–12, 129–133, 257–260.

Purkinje, J. E. (1865, in Czech). Man's individual mental mechanism. *Krok, 2*, 1–5.

Purkinje, J. E. (1867). *Austria polyglotta* (in Czech and in German), Prague.

Purkinje, J. E. (1918). *Opera omnia* (Vol. 1). (K. J. Lhotak, Ed.). Prague: Society of Czech Physicians.

Purkinje, J. E. (1937). *Opera omnia* (Vol. 2). (F. K. Studnička, Ed.). Prague: State Health Publishing House.

Purkinje, J. E. (1939). *Opera omnia* (Vol. 3). (F. K. Studnička, Ed.). Prague: State Health Publishing House.

Purkinje, J. E. (1941). *Opera omnia* (Vol. 4). (F. K. Studnička, Ed.). Prague: State Health Publishing House.

Purkinje, J. E. (1948). *Opera selecta* (Z. Frankenberger, K. Hübschmann, F. Karasek, V. Kruta, V. Laufberger, and F. K. Studnička, Eds.). Prague. Association of Czech Medical Men.
Purkinje, J. E. (1951). *Opera omnia* (Vol. 5). (V. Kruta and Z. Hornof, Eds.). Prague: State Health Publishing House.
Purkinje, J. E. (1954). *Opera omnia* (Vol. 6). (V. Kruta and Z. Hornof, Eds.). Prague: State Health Publishing House.
Purkinje, J. E. (1958). *Opera omnia* (Vol. 7). (B. Nemec, Ed.). Prague: Academia.
Purkinje, J. E. (1960). *Opera omnia* (Vol. 8). (V. Kruta and Z. Hornof, Eds.). Prague: Academia.
Purkinje, J. E. (1965). *Opera omnia* (Vol. 9). (V. Kruta and Z. Hornof, Eds.). Prague: Academia.
Purkinje, J. E. (1968). *Opera omnia* (Vol. 10). (M. Kudelk, ed.). Prague: Academia.
Purkinje, J. E. (1968). *Opera omnia* (Vol. 11). (J. Thon, ed.). Prague: Academia.
Purkinje, J. E. (1969). *Opera omnia* (Vol. 12). (V. Kruta, ed.). Prague: Academia.
Purkinje, J. E. (1985). *Opera omnia* (Vol. 13). (V. Kruta and V. Zapletal, Eds.). Prague: Academia.
Ratliff, F. (1971). On the objective study of subjective phenomena: The Purkyně tree. In V. Kruta (Ed.), *Jan Evangelista Purkyně 1787–1869. Centenary symposium* (pp. 77–92). Brno, Czechoslovakia: Universita Jana Evangelisty Purkyně.
Reid, T. (1764). *An inquiry into the human mind, on the principles of common sense*. Edinburgh: Millar, Kincaid & Bell.
Rieger, F. L. (1867, in Czech). Jan Evangelista Purkinje. *Dictionary* (Vol. 6, pp. 1115–1119). Prague: Kober.
Ritter, J. W. (1801). Versuche und Bemerkungen über den Galvanismus der Voltaischen Batterie. *Annalen der Physik*, *7*, 431–484.
Ritter, J. W. (1805). Neue Versuche und Bemerkungen über den Galvanismus. *Annalen der Physik*, *19*, 1–54.
Rohault, J. (1671). *Traité de physique*. Paris: Savreux.
Rose, F. C. & Bynum, W. F. (Eds.). (1982). *Historical aspects of the neurosciences. A Festschrift for Macdonald Critchley*. New York: Raven.
Rosen, E. (1956a). The invention of eyeglasses. *Journal of the History of Medicine*, *11*, 13–46.
Rosen, E. (1956b). The invention of eyeglasses. *Journal of the History of Medicine*, *11*, 183–218.
Ross, W. D. (Ed.). (1913). *The works of Aristotle* (Vol. 6). Oxford, England: Clarendon.
Ross, W. D. (Ed.). (1927). *The works of Aristotle* (Vol. 7). Oxford, England: Clarendon.
Ross, W. D. (Ed.). (1931). *The works of Aristotle* (Vol. 3). Oxford, England: Clarendon.
Rothschuh, K. E. (1973). *History of physiology*. (G. B. Risse, Trans.). Huntington, NY: Krieger.
Sabra, A. I. (Trans. and ed.). (1989). *The Optics of Ibn Al-Haytham. Books I–III. On direct vision*. London: The Warburg Institute.
Sahakian, W. S. (1968). *History of psychology. A sourcebook of systematic psychology* (pp. 101–108). Itasca, IL: P. E. Peacock.
Sanson, L. J. (1838). *Leçons sur la maladies des yeux*. Paris: Bardinot and Pigne.
Scheiner, C. (1619). *Oculus, hoc est fundamentum opticum*. Innsbruck, Austria: Agricola.
Scherffer, K. (1761). *De coloribus accidentalibus*. Vienna: Trattner.
Schmitz, E.-H. (1982). *Handbuch zur Geschichte der Optik* (Vol. 2). Bonn: Wayerborgh.
Schmitz, E.-H. (1995). *Handbuch zur Geschichte der Optik* (Supplementary Vol. 3). Bonn: Wayerborgh.
Schwann, T. (1839). *Mikroskopische Untersuchungen über die Übereinstimmung in der Struktur und dem Wachsthum der Tiere und Pflanzen*. Berlin: Reimer.
Seneca. (63/1971). *Naturales quaestiones* (T. H. Corcoran, Trans.). London: Heinemann.
Shastid, T. H. (1917). History of ophthalmology. In C. A. Wood, (Ed.), *The American encyclopedia and dictionary of ophthalmology* (Vol. 11, pp. 8524–8904). Chicago: Cleveland Press.
Shepherd, G. (1991). *Foundations of the neuron doctrine*. New York: Oxford University Press.
Sherrington, C. S. (1906). *The integrative action of the nervous system*. New Haven: Yale University Press.

Shryock, R. H. (1944). The strange case of Wells' theory of natural selection. In M. F. A. Montagu, (Ed.), *Studies and essays in the history of science and learning offered in homage to George Sarton* (pp. 197–207). New York: Schuman.

Singer, C. (1921). Steps leading to the invention of the first optical apparatus. In C. Singer, (Ed.), *Studies in the history and method of science* (pp. 385–413). Oxford: Clarendon.

Smith, A. M. (1996). *Ptolemy's theory of visual perception: An English translation of the* Optics *with introduction and commentary*. Philadelphia: The American Philosophical Society.

Smith, R. (1738). *A compleat system of opticks in four books*. Cambridge: Published for the author.

Smith, R. (1755). *Vollständiger Lehrbegriff der Optik* (A. G. Kästner, Trans.). Altenburg, Germany: Richter.

Smythies, J. R. (1957). A preliminary analysis of the stroboscopic patterns. *Nature (London) 179*, 523–524.

Soemmerring, S. T. von. (1801). *Abbildungen des menschlichen Auges*. Frankfurt: Varrentrapp and Wenner.

Spillane, J. D. (1981). *The doctrine of the nerves*. Oxford, England: Oxford University Press.

Stampfer, S. (1833). *Die stroboskopischen Scheiben oder optische Zauberscheiben, deren Theorie und Wissenschaftliche Anwendung*. Vienna: Trentsensky & Vieweg.

Steinbuch, J. G. (1811). *Beytrag zur Physiologie der Sinne*. Nürnberg, Germany: Schrag.

Stratton, G. M. (1917). *Theophrastus and the Greek physiological psychology before Aristotle*. New York: Macmillan.

Talbot, H. F. (1834). Experiments on light. *The London and Edinburgh Philosophical Magazine and Journal of Science, 5*, 321–334.

Thompson, R. F. (Ed.). (1986). *Progress in neuroscience*. New York: Freeman.

Thomsen, E. (1919). Über Johannes Evangelista Purkinje und seine Werke. Purkinjes entoptische Phänomene. Auf Basis biographischer Daten und anderer Untersuchungen. *Skandanavisches Archiv für Physiologie, 37*, 1–116.

Tourtual, C. T. (1827). *Die Sinne des Menschen in den wechselseitigen Beziehungen ihres psychischen und organischen Lebens*. Muenster, Germany: Regensberg.

Troxler, D. (1804). Ueber das Verschwinden gegebener Gegenstände innerhalb unseres Gesichtskreises. *Ophthalmologische Bibliothek, 2*, 1–53.

Turnbull, H. W. (Ed.) (1960). *The correspondence of Isaac Newton, Volume 2. 1676–1687*. Cambridge, England: Cambridge University Press.

Valentin, G. G. (1836). Über den Verlauf und die letzten Ende der Nerven. *Nova Acta Physico-Medica Academae Caesarae Leopoldina-Carolinae Naturae Curiosorum, 18*, 51–240.

Vavroušek, B., Hykeš, O. V., & Noval, A. (1937, in Czech). *Album Jana Ev. Purkyně*. Prague: Prometheus.

Votava, Z. (1971). Purkyně's pioneer contribution to neuro-psychopharmacology. In V. Kruta (Ed.), *Jan Evangelista Purkyně 1787–1869. Centenary symposium* (pp. 47–55). Brno, Czechoslovakia: Universita Jana Evangelisty Purkyně.

Wade, N. J. (1977a). A note on the discovery of subjective colours. *Vision Research, 17*, 671–672.

Wade, N. J. (1977b). Distortions and disappearances of geometrical patterns. *Perception, 6*, 407–433.

Wade, N. J. (1978a). Why do patterned afterimages fluctuate in visibility? *Psychological Bulletin, 85*, 338–352.

Wade, N. J. (1978b). Sir Charles Bell on visual direction. *Perception, 7*, 359–362.

Wade, N. (1982). *The art and science of visual illusions*. London: Routledge & Kegan Paul.

Wade, N. J., (Ed.). (1983). *Brewster and Wheatstone on vision*. London: Academic.

Wade, N. J. (1987). On the late invention of the stereoscope. *Perception, 16*, 785–818.

Wade, N. (1990). *Visual allusions: Pictures of perception*. Hove, East Sussex, England: Lawrence Erlbaum Associates.

Wade, N. J. (1994). A selective history of the study of visual motion aftereffects. *Perception, 23*, 1111–1134.

Wade, N. J. (1998a). *A natural history of vision.* Cambridge, MA.: MIT Press.
Wade, N. J. (1998b). Early studies of eye dominances. *Laterality, 3*, 97–109.
Wade, N. J. (1998c). Light and sight since antiquity. *Perception, 27*, 637–670.
Wade, N. (1998d). Illusions as neuro-signs. *Current Biology, 8*, R364–365.
Wade, N. J. (2000a). Porterfield and Wells on the motions of our eyes. *Perception, 29*, 221–239.
Wade, N. J. (2000b). Jean Théophile Desaguliers (1683–1744) and eighteenth century vision research. *British Journal of Psychology, 91*, 275–285.
Wade, N. J. (2000c). William Charles Wells (1757–1817) and vestibular research before Purkinje and Flourens. *Journal of Vestibular Research, 10*, 127–137.
Wade, N. J. (Ed.) (2000d). *The Emergence of neuroscience in the nineteenth century.* (8 Vols.). London: Routledge.
Wade, N. J., & Heller, D. (1997). Scopes of perception: The experimental manipulation of space and time. *Psychological Research, 60*, 227–237.
Wade, N. J., & Verstraten, F. A. J. (1998). Introduction and historical overview. In G. Mather, F. Verstraten, and S. Anstis, (Eds.), *The motion after-effect: A modern perspective* (pp. 1–23). Cambridge, MA: MIT Press.
Wardrop, J. (1808). *Essays on the morbid anatomy of the human eye* (Vol. 1). Edinburgh: Archibald Constable.
Wardrop, J. (1818). *Essays on the morbid anatomy of the human eye* (Vol. 2). Edinburgh: Archibald Constable.
Wells, W. C. (1792). *An essay upon single vision with two eyes: together with experiments and observations on several other subjects in optics.* London: Cadell.
Wells, W. C. (1794a). Reply to Dr. Darwin on vision. *The Gentleman's Magazine and Historical Chronicle, 64*, 794–797.
Wells, W. C. (1794b). Reply to Dr. Darwin on vision. *The Gentleman's Magazine and Historical Chronicle, 64*, 905–907.
Wells, W. C. (1811). Observations and experiments on vision. *Philosophical Transactions of the Royal Society, 101*, 378–391.
Wells, C. (1813). Beobachtungen und Versuche über das Sehen. *Annalen der Physik, 43*, 128–143.
Wells, W. C. (1818). *Two essays: One upon single vision with two eyes; the other on dew.* London: Constable.
Wetzel, K. (1800). *Grundriss der eigenlichen Systems der anthropologischen Psychologie überhaupt and der empirischen insbesondere.* (Vol. 1). Leipzig: Dyck.
Wetzel, K. (1805). *Grundriss der eigenlichen Systems der anthropologischen Psychologie überhaupt and der empirischen insbesondere.* (Vol. 2). Leipzig: Dyck.
Wheatstone, C. (1827). Description of the kaleidophone, or phonic kaleidoscope; A new philosophical toy, for the illustration of several interesting and amusing acoustical and optical phenomena. *Quarterly Journal of Science, Literature and Art, 23*, 344–351.
Wheatstone, C. (1838). Contributions to the physiology of vision—Part the first. On some remarkable, and hitherto unobserved, phenomena of binocular vision. *Philosophical Transactions of the Royal Society, 128*, 371–394.
Whytt, R. (1763). *An essay on the vital and other involuntary motions of animals* (2nd ed.). Edinburgh: Hamilton, Balfour, and Neill.
Whytt, R. (1765). *Observations on the nature, causes, and cure of those disorders which have commonly been called nervous hypochondriac, or hysteric.* Edinburgh: Becket, Du Hondt, and Balfour.
Wilkins, A. J. (1995). *Visual stress.* New York: Oxford University Press.
Willis, T. (1664). *Cerebri anatome: cui accessit nervorum descriptio et usus.* London: Martyn and Allestry.
Willis, T. (1672). *De anima brutorum.* London: Wells & Scott.
Wood, C. A. (1929). *Benevenutus Grassus of Jerusalem De Oculis.* Stanford: Stanford University Press.

Young, T. (1793). Observations on vision. *Philosophical Transactions of the Royal Society, 83*, 169–181.

Young, T. (1800). Outlines of experiments and enquiries respecting sound and light. *Philosophical Transactions of the Royal Society, 90*, 106–150.

Young, T. (1801). On the mechanism of the eye. *Philosophical Transactions of the Royal Society, 91*, 23–88.

Young, T. (1802). On the theory of lights and colours. *Philosophical Transactions of the Royal Society, 92*, 12–48.

Zeki, S. (1999). *Inner vision. An exploration of art and the brain.* Oxford, England: Oxford University Press.

Zeki, S., Watson, J. D. G., & Frackowiak, R. S. J. (1993). Going beyond the information given: The relation of illusory visual motion to brain activity. *Proceedings of the Royal Society of London, Series B, 252*, 215–222.

Name Index

Ægineta, P., 10
Aguilonius, F., 52, 59
Alcmaeon, 44
Alhazen, (see also Ibn al-Haytham), 11
Anstis, S., 15
Arens, K., 13
Ariotti, P. E., 52
Aristotle, 8, 10, 14–16, 48, 53, 60, 113
Armati, S., 10
Aubert, H., 23

Bacon, F., 48
Bacon, R., 9, 59
Bárány, R., 17
Barlow, H. B., 122
Bartisch, G., 10
Bell, C., 10, 11, 19, 50, 61, 123
Bender, M. B., 118
Berkeley, G., 27, 37
Bernoulli, J., 82
Boerhaave, H., 57
Boring, E. G., 17, 22
Boulton, M., 18
Brazier, M. A. B., 26, 46, 114
Breuer, J., 22, 23
Brewster, D., 49, 104, 112, 125
Brindley, G., 122
Brown, A. Crum, 22
Brown, J. L., 124
Brožek, J., xii, xiii, 13, 14, 26, 27, 33, 35–37, 66
Buffon, Comte de, 52
Burdach, K. F., 33, 39
Burke, R. B., 59
Burton, H. E., 11
Bynum, W. F., 26

C.W., 51, 58, 115, 119, 125
Cahan, D., 115
Caliandro, M., xiii
Castelli, B., 52
Chladni, E. F. F., 31, 75
Clarke, E., 25, 26, 114
Cohen, B., 20
Cohen, J., 121
Comenius, J. A., 29
Cox, J. M., 18
Cramer, A., 113
Crombie, A. C., 8
Cutting, Dr., 7

Dallenbach, K. M., 121
D'Arcy, Chevalier, 54
Darwin, C., 19
Darwin, E., 4, 15–21, 49, 55, 62, 117, 118
Darwin, R. W., 19, 20, 52–54, 57, 60, 61, 117
de Lepinay, J., 13
Desaguliers, J. T., 5, 47, 119, 120
Descartes, R., 5, 10, 45, 119, 120
Dewhurst, K., 15
Dietrichstein, Cardinal, 30
Diogenes Laertius, 16
Donders, F. C., 7, 112
Dostalek, K. C., 37
Du Tour, E.-F., 47
Duke-Elder, S., 10
Dusser de Barenne, J. G., 17

Ehrenberg, C. G., 37
Eichel, J., 58, 100
Elliott, J., 45, 58, 100, 101, 119
Emmert, E., 52

Erb, M. B., 121
Euclid, 11
Euler, L., 82

Fancher, R. E., 22
Fechner, G. T., 51, 121, 122
Ferrier, D., 114
Fichte, J. G., 27, 30
Finger, S., 26, 46, 114
Flourens, M. J. P., 15–17, 21–23, 33, 38, 39, 116–118
Frackowiak, R. S. J., 56
Franklin, B., 10, 53
Franz, S. I., 51
Fritz, I., 31, 32

Galen, C., 10, 59, 61, 114
Gall, F. J., 21, 22, 62, 111, 114
Galvani, L., 46, 114
Goethe, J. W., 2, 4, 27, 42, 45, 48, 115, 118, 121
Gordon, D. A., 121
Grassus, B., 57
Gray, A. A., 23
Griffith, C. R., 16, 17
Gruithuisen, F., 116
Grüsser, O.-J., 2, 4, 17, 18, 44
Gwei-Djen, L., 8

Hagner, M., 44
Hallaran, W. S., 18
Harris, J., 11, 12, 48, 60
Hartley, D., 11
Hatfield, G., 4, 26
Heller, D., 3
Helmholtz, H., 2, 5, 41, 42, 47, 58, 61, 112, 113, 122, 126
Henn, V., 22, 23
Herbart, J. F., 33
Hering, E., 27, 47
Herrnstein, R. J., 22
Herz, M., 17
Hildprandt, F., 31, 32
Hill, E., 8
Himly, K., 84
Hirschberg, J., 10
Home, E., 100
Hooke, R., 24
Hoskovec, J., xii, 26, 27, 33, 35–37, 39, 66
Howard, I. P., 22, 58
Hume, D., 3, 27
Hykeš, O. V., 110, 127

Ibn al-Haytham, 11, 12, 48, 54, 59
Ilg, J. G., 31

John, H. J., 8, 9, 12, 34
Judd, D. B., 52
Jurin, J., 10, 11, 48, 54, 59

Kant, I., 3, 27, 30, 33
Kästner, A. G., 84
Kepler, J., 3, 5, 10, 48
King-Hele, D., 18
Klemm, O., 113
Klotz, M., 14, 113
Koelbing, H. M., 57
Kornhuber, H. H., 15
Kotek, V., 29, 32
Krauss, H. C. G., 38, 116
Kruta, V., 2, 16, 17, 21, 23–25, 39, 42, 65, 115, 116
Kuthan, V., 13

La Hire, P. de, 5, 50, 57, 123, 124
Le Clerc, S., 47
Leeuwenhoek, A. van, 24
Leonardo da Vinci, 14, 54, 113
Lhotak, K. J., 34
Liddell, E. G., 25, 26
Locke, J., 27, 62
Lotze, R. H., 33
Lucretius, T. C., 15, 16

MacCurdy, E., 54
Mach, E., 15, 22, 23
Mariotte, E., 48–50, 60, 82, 86, 122
Mather, G., 15, 24
Matousek, O., 43
Maurolico, F., 10
May, M. T., 10, 59, 61
McHenry, L. C., 26
McKendrick, J. G., 23
Mile, J., 115
Minnaert, M., 113
Morgagni, J. B., 45
Moritz, K. P., 33
Müller, H., 124
Müller, J., 15, 22, 33, 37, 39, 115, 118, 122

Needham, J., 8
Newton, I., 2, 3, 45, 52–54, 59, 69, 92, 119, 121
Nicati, W., 13
Niklicek, L., 29, 32
Noval, A., 127
Novalis, (F. von Hardenberg), 31

O'Malley, C. D., 25, 26, 114
Ono, H., 61

Paré, A., 10
Park, D., 3, 44
Pecham, J., 48
Pecquet, A., 50, 122
Pestalozzi, J. H., 31
Picard, 84
Piccolono, M., 46, 114
Plateau, J., 43, 115
Platter, F., 48, 57
Pliny the Elder, 7, 8
Pohl, J. E., 31
Porta, J. B., 47, 59
Porterfield, W., 5, 6, 17–20, 60
Priestley, J., 5, 18, 19, 54
Prochaska, G., 114
Psotníčková, J., 27, 32, 43, 63
Ptolemy, C., 11, 12, 16, 53, 54, 58, 59
Purkinje, Josef, 29
Purkinje, Rosalie, 29

Quetelet, A., 33

Ratliff, F., 124
Reid, T., 10, 11, 27, 47
Rieger, F. L., 30, 31
Ritter, J. W., 46, 122
Rogers, B., 58
Rohault, J., 5
Rose, F. C., 26
Rosen, E., 8, 10
Ross, W. D., 8, 10, 60, 113
Rothschuh, K. E., 27, 35, 115
Rottenberger, J., 31
Rudolphi, K. A., 35, 39
Rudolphi, J., 35
Rust, J. V., 32

Sabra, A. I., 11, 12, 59
Safranek, R., 29
Sahakian, W. S., 34
Sanson, L. J., 113
Scheiner, C., 3, 5, 44, 48, 56, 60
Schelling, F. W. J. von, 27, 30
Scherffer, K., 53
Schmid, J., 65
Schmidt, F., 31
Schmidt, J. A., 84
Schmitz, E.-H., 8, 10
Schwann, T., 24, 25
Seebek, A., 86, 89
Seneca, 8, 53
Shanzer, S., 118
Shastid, T. H., 10
Shepherd, G., 26
Sherrington, C. S., 26, 114, 115
Shryock, R. H., 117
Singer, C., 8
Smith, A. M., 11, 54
Smith, R., 49, 59, 84
Smythies, J. R., 42
Soemmerring, S. T. von, 51
Spillane, J. D., 26
Spurzheim, J. C., 62
Stampfer, S., 43
Steinbuch, J. G., 4, 5, 96, 119
Stratton, G. M., 44

Talbot, H. F., 122
Templeton, W. B., 22
Theophrastus, 16
Thompson, R., 23
Thomsen, E., 16, 24
Tommaso da Modena, 10
Tourtual, C. T., 34, 35, 37, 39
Troxler, D., 49, 84, 86
Turnbull, H. W., 59

Valentin, G. G., 24, 25
Vavroušek, B., 127
Verstraten, F., 15
Volta, A., 46, 122
Votava, Z., 26, 113

Wade, N. J., xiii, 3, 6, 10, 14–16, 20, 26, 44, 48, 51, 53, 55, 56, 58, 61, 62, 114, 117, 119–121, 124
Wagner, R., 36, 38
Wardrop, J., 112
Watson, J. D. G., 56
Watt, J., 18

Wawruch, A., 31, 32
Wedgwood, J., 18
Wells, W. C., 6, 7, 16, 17, 19–21, 23, 59, 61, 62, 117–119, 126
Wetzel, K., 33
Wheatstone, C., 51, 54, 58, 115, 118, 119, 122, 125
Whytt, R., 16, 37, 56
Wilkins, A., 55
Wilkinson, E., xii
Willis, T., 15–17, 21, 22, 57
Wood, C. A., 57
Wybar, K., 10

Young, T., 2, 6, 12, 45, 49, 50, 54, 60, 112, 113, 126

Zeki, S., 56, 124

Subject Index

A

aberrations, 126
ablation, 22
Academia, 33
accelerations of the head, 22
accidental colors, 2, 51–53
accommodation, 5–10, 34, 42, 60, 120
  cloudy streaks and, 55
  coining of term, 5
  effects of belladonna on, 7, 8, 12, 26, 119
  Helmholtz and, 5, 113
  lens involvement in, 6, 7, 113
  mechanism of, 5–7, 113
  optometer and, 6
  Priestley's view, 5
  pupil constriction and, 5, 56
  Purkinje images and, 5, 112
  theories of, 5
achromatic lens, 113
achromatic microscope, 2, 24, 35, 113
Achromatopsia, 39
acoustic movement, 76
acoustics, 54
action potentials, 114
acuity, 60
afferent signals, 61
aftereffect of seen movement, 15
aftereffects, 42, 124
afterimage, 20, 42, 51–54, 67, 121, 124
  apparent size of, 52
  as stabilized retinal image, 51, 61, 126
  color sequence in, 53, 72, 89–92, 124
  colored, 52, 89–92
  duration of visibility, 53, 90, 124
  fixation and, 60, 105
  fluctuations, 52, 89, 91, 107
  foveal, 51
  interocular transfer of, 52
  latency, 53
  motion of, 19, 61
  negative, 51–53, 91
  patterned, 52, 91
  peripheral, 61
  persisting images and, 62, 107
  positive, 51–53, 91
  primary stimulus, 52
  Purkinje's description of, 88–92
  Purkyně's phase, 124
  retinal blood vessel figure and, 91
  second positive phase, 52, 124
  spectra and, 117
  Troxler effect and, 49
  vertigo and, 17
alcohol, 81, 107
  as fixative, 25
  vertigo and, 16, 17
altars, 106
alternating dominance, 47
alternating illumination, 69, 70
amativeness, 22
amblyopia, 11
American Psychological Association, 37
ampulla, 22
analogy, 68, 75
anatomical specimens, 24
anatomy, 31, 115
angular acceleration, 22, 23
angular velocity, 23
animal cells, 24
animal electricity, 114
animal eyes, 102
animal instincts, 36
animal species, 87

animal spirit, 16, 17, 21–23, 46, 114
anisotropy, 126
anode, 46
antagonistic eye muscles, 105
anthropological psychology, 33
antiquity, 3, 4, 16, 44, 46, 48, 114
anti-reticularists, 26
aphakia, 6
apparent distance, 120
apparent motion, 14, 16, 17, 21, 43, 61, 125
apparent rotation, 20
apparent size, 120
aqueous humor, 57, 113
aristocratic taste, 106
art, 106
art and science, 2
arterial system, 77
artists, 115, 124
association, 4, 39
associationist theory, 5, 62
asthenia, 107
astigmatism, 47, 50, 126
  transient, 56
astronomical apparatus, 30
astronomy, 29
asylums for the insane, 18
atmosphere, 82
attention, 82, 104
  afterimage visibility and, 52
  fixing, 13, 61
  fluctuations of, 81
auditory localization, 22
auricular murmurs, 21
Austria Polyglotta, 36
Austrian empire, 36
Autognosie, 36
autopsies, 31
axis
  of eye, 20, 60, 78, 83, 103
  of head, 21
  of vision, 11, 49–51, 59
  optic, 48, 83, 84

B

balance, 16, 21
Barbadoes, 7
beauty, 76
Beiträge zur Kenntniss des Sehens in subjectiver Hinsicht, 2, 4, 64, 119
belladonna, 12, 26, 34, 119
  accommodation and, 7, 8, 26, 113
Beobachtungen über die Sinne, 119
Beobachtungen und Versuche zur Physiologie der Sinne, 4, 64
Berkeley's theory of vision, 37
Berlin, 115
Beytrag zur Physiologie der Sinne, 4, 119
Bidwell's ghost, 124
bifocal glasses, 10
binocular correspondence, 58, 59
binocular rivalry, 47, 59, 122
binocular vision, 10, 119, 120, 122
  and direction, 59, 117
  blind spot in, 83
  Purkinje's description of, 102–104
  singleness of, 11, 42, 58, 59, 122
  stereoscopic, 58, 59
  theories of, 59
biological sciences, 24
biology, 111
birds, 22
Blatna, 31
Blendungsbilder, 51, 62, 124
blind people, 46, 106
blind spot, 42, 48–50, 83, 123
  diagram of, 83
  Purkinje's description of, 82–86
  visibility around, 122
blinding images, 124
blinding the eyes, 89
blindness, temporary, 48
blinking, 62, 107
blood circulation in eye
  diagram of, 96
  visibility of, 42, 67
blood corpuscles, 96
blood supply, 74, 76
blood vessels, 77
blood-vessel pattern (*see also* Purkinje tree), 73, 74
body movement, 107
body position, 15, 23
body rotation, 14, 16–18, 20, 23, 43, 44
body tilt, 23
Bohemia, xii, 29–31
botany, 31, 67
brain, 39, 62, 77, 108, 113
  abnormalities in, 114
  activity, 124
  and spinal cord, 25

development, 23
functions of, 111, 124
gross anatomy of, 114
imaging, 24, 56, 124
motion of, 21, 22
pressure in, 18
Purkinje cells in, 1
recording, 24
relation to vertigo, 16–18, 116
structure, 23
substance, 114
Breslau, 2, 5, 12, 33–38, 111
institute of experimental physiology, 115
medical school, 35
brightness contrast, 14
British empiricists, 27
Brockhaus Enzyklopädie, 14
burning glass, 8

C

camera, 3
camphor, 26
carotids, 74, 76
cascade, 21
cataract, 7, 82, 113
cathartics, 18
cathode, 46
cavalry parade, 14
cell, 35, 38, 76, 114
descriptions of, xi
doctrine, 24, 114
histology, 37
periphery, 114
Purkinje, xi, 1, 2, 25, 113
structure, 37, 38, 115
theory, 2, 25, 114
Central Europe, 115
central vision, 50
cerebellar lesions, 17, 22, 116, 117
cerebellum, xi, 21, 22, 24, 116, 117
cerebral affectations, 107
cerebral hemispheres, 25
cerebral ischemia, 17
cerebral localization, 21, 22, 56, 62, 111
cerebral ventricles, 114
cerebrum, 117
chaotic light, 79
Charles University, xii
checkerboard pattern, 42, 46, 69, 74
chemical science, 111
chemical transmission, 26, 115
chemist, 67
chemistry, 33, 115
chess board, 69
child, 68
childhood, 36
Chladni figures, 31, 75
choroid, 50, 86, 87
chromatic aberration, 8
chronoscope, 3, 115
ciliary motion, 38
ciliary muscles, 56, 113
ciliary process, 6, 57
clothes, 106
clouds, 82
cloudy streaks, 47, 49, 67, 84, 92
afterimages and, 93, 94
Purkinje's description of, 92–94
clowns, 106
cognitive dysfunction, 114
color, 4, 27, 34, 121
blindness, 2, 113
brightness of, 1, 34
combination, 14, 34
contrast, 2, 80
differences between individuals, 113
differences within individuals, 12
discrimination, 12
disk, 53, 54
experience, 2, 4, 121
game, 90
mixing, 2–4
phenomena, 3
rivalry, 47
shadows, 2
theory, 2, 14, 67
top, 53, 92
zones, 12, 13
comets, 53
Commentatio, 37
common axis, 59
comparative physiology, 118
complementary aftereffect, 56
complementary afterimages, 52
Comprehensive Theory of Colors, 14
concave lens, 50, 93
concentric circles, 55, 56, 93
conditioned responses, 37
conductors, 77, 78
cones, 1

conjunctiva, 46
conscious movements, 117
consciousness, 39, 77, 103
loss of, 77
unity of, 103, 108
Contributions to the knowledge of vision in its subjective aspects, 2, 41, 66, 119
Contributions to the Physiology of the Senses, 4
convergence, 83
convergent strabismus, 11
convex glass, 82
copper engravings, 55, 92, 93
copper pole, 46, 77, 78
cornea, 113
curvature of, 6, 112
pressure on, 71, 104
reflections from, 5, 8, 9, 112
cortical localization, 21, 22, 56, 62, 111
coughing, 99
cranial nerves, 114
cranioscopy, 39
creative genius, 106
crystalline lens (*see also* lens), 99, 100, 112
as receptive organ, 10
flying gnats and, 97
light dispersion and, 94
visual patterns and, 76, 77
crystallization, 79
curvilinear star pattern, 67
diagram of, 98
Purkinje's description of, 98, 99
Cyklus der physiologischen Doktrinen, 33
Czech language, xii
Czech National Academy of Sciences, 33
Czech patriotism, xi
Czech science, xii

D

dance, 106
dark adaptation, 48
dark field, 47, 80–82
dawn, 1, 13
daylight, 48
daze, 105
deaf, 46
deception, 19
decorations, 106
deep breathing, 75, 76
desire, 33
Dictionary of Physiology, 36
digestion, 39
digitalis, 26, 34
direct sensory perception, 108
direct vision, 11–13, 34
disappearance, 49, 66
disease, 4, 17
distance vision, 34
distinct vision, 55, 60, 93, 125
limits of, 6, 10
peripheral and, 11, 12
vertigo and, 15
distraction, 104
divergent strabismus, 11
dizziness, 14–17, 19
double refraction, 104
double vision, 10, 42, 58, 59, 67
monocular, 104
Purkinje's description of, 102–104
drawing, 71, 77, 93
dreams, 36, 67, 109
drives, 36
drugs, 26, 116
self-administered, xi, 26, 32, 113
dusk, 1, 13, 14, 48, 113

E

Ebers papyrus, 10
education, 106
educational reform, 38
efferent impulses, 61
effort, strenuous, 74
egg yolk, 37, 111
Eigengrau, 47
eight-ray star, 73
elasticity, 39, 76
electrical current, 114
electrical discharges, 46, 77, 79, 85
electrical stimulation, 17, 46, 121
electricity, 6, 46, 86, 108, 114
electrodes, 46, 78, 79, 122
emetine, 37
emission theories of light, 44
Emmert's law, 52
emotions, 36
empirical knowledge, 68
empirical psychology, xii, 26, 27, 33, 35, 67
empiricism, 5, 27

empiricist philosophers, 3
Encyclopädisches Wörterbuch der medicinischen Wissenschaften, 38
endolymph, 22
endurance, 77
English, 35, 65
engraving, 93, 94, 122, 125
entoptic phenomena, 42, 57, 58, 86, 123
environment, natural, 3
epileptic seizures, 117
equilibrium, 22, 105
errors of refraction, 8
Erzeugung, 39
Essay upon Single Vision with Two Eyes, 59, 117
exact subjectivism, 24, 26, 115
existence, 67
experience, 2, 4
  physiology and, 4, 24
  subjective, 1, 4, 88, 116
  world of, 68
experimental methods, 111
experimental physiology, 115, 116
experimental science, 115
external world, 68
extirpation, 22
extraocular muscles, 61
eye
  activity of, 107
  anatomy of, 3, 10
  artificial, 3
  camera and, 3
  corrections, 8
  dioptrics of, 10
  dominance, 59
  excitability of, 74
  image movement and, 61
  nervous core of, 76
  optical surfaces of, 1
  perceptual activity of, 106
  position, 15, 61
  rotations, 17, 20, 61, 105
  sense of feeling in, 107
  sense of touch and, 106
  socket, 101, 105
  spatial activity of, 107
  visual axis of, 8
eye movements, 42, 49, 60–62, 67
  anisotropies of, 126
  circular patterns and, 105
  delicate, 106
  horizontal, 105
  in the blind, 60
  in the feeble-minded, 60, 106
  involuntary, 61, 62
  language of, 106
  Müller's research, 118
  observation of, 126
  postrotary, 17, 19–21, 61, 126
  posture and, 22
  Purkinje's descriptions of, 105–106
  Purkinje's research on, 121, 126
  rotating patterns and, 92
  unconscious, 14, 15, 17
  vertical, 105
  voluntary, 60–62
  Wells' account of, 61, 62
eyeball, 98–101, 106
eyeglasses, 8, 10
eyelids, 62, 70, 72, 78, 85, 98
  closure of, 107
eyes
  as separate entities, 103
  deviations of, 10, 11
  differences between, 104
  separation of, 103

F

faculty psychology, 33
fainting, 74, 76
fantasy, 67, 76
far point of vision, 6, 7, 10
Farbenlehre, 2
fatigue, 80
Fechner colors, 121
feeling, 33
fever, 18, 97
fingerprints, xi, 111
  diagram of, 112
fireworks, 106
firey rings, 58, 79, 92, 102
fixation, 67, 79, 93–95
  on targets, 49, 60
  point, 59, 104
flicker, 81, 85, 121
  methods of producing, 42
  of candle flame, 69
  patterns, 71, 121
fliegende Mücken, 57
floaters, 50, 57, 123, 124

Florence, 10
fluctuating light, 73
fluctuations of visibility, 84
flying gnats (*see also* floaters), 57, 67, 123
  blood corpuscles and, 97
  diagram of, 97
  Purkinje's description of, 96–98
folly, 108
forensic scientists, xi
fovea, 51, 124
free will, 2
French, 30, 65
friction machines, 46
frost, 74

G

Galvani's experiments, 46, 114
galvanic light figures, 34, 46, 66, 101, 122
  and light and shade figures, 76
  diagram of, 78
  Purkinje's description of, 77–79
  scintillations and, 47
  secondary forms, 79
galvanic stimulation, 17, 42, 75, 80, 87, 122
Galvanism, 6
games, 69
ganglia, 114
ganglion cells, 124
ganglionic corpuscles, 114
Ganzfeld, 47
gardens, 106
Gentleman's Magazine, 117
geography, 30
geometrical patterns, 56, 106, 124
German philosophers, 29, 30
germinal vesicle, 37, 111
giddiness (*see also* vertigo), 16, 20
Glance at Contemporary Psychology, 37
glare figures (*see* afterimages), 89
glass lens, 86
glass plate, 75
Goethe, 2
  influence on Purkinje, 2, 42, 121
  phenomenology of, 2
  review of Purkinje's dissertation, 118
  vision research, 4, 42, 45, 48
gratings, 124
gravity, 23
gray matter, 24
Greek, 29, 30
ground-glass lenses, 8
Gründliche Farbenlehre, 14
Grundlinien der Zergliederungskunde des menschlichen Körpers, 31
guitar strings, 77, 79
gymnasium, 30
gymnastics, 106

H

haemophthalmus, 98
halos, 49, 50, 66
  Purkinje's description of, 87
Handbuch der Physiologie des Menschen, 22
Handwörterbuch der Physiologie, 36
harmony of the organism, 109
head movement, 17, 21, 49
head position, 19, 21
head rotation, 22
head, emptiness of, 104
health, 4
hearing, 15, 21, 22
heart, xi, 1, 16, 18, 113
heart, pumping action of, 43, 44
heautognostisch, 26
hexagons, 69, 73, 77
histologists, xi
histology, 38, 39
  cradle of, 2
History of Psychology Newsletter, 37
History of Psychology, 34
history, 30, 36, 119, 126
  of light and vision, 19
  of the senses, 15
  of the vestibular system, 118
  of vision, xii, 44
  of visual science, 122
honey, 7
horizon, 23
horopter, 59
human condition, 106
Human Senses with Reference to Mutual Relations of Psychological and Organic Processes, 34–35
hydrodynamic theory of vestibular function, 23
hyperopia, 47
hypochondria, 88
hysteria, 88

I

Ibn al-Haytham's board, 11, 12, 59
idealism, 27
illusions, 41, 67
image formation, 3, 48, 86
imagination, 62, 67, 106, 108
  blind spot and, 49
  faculty psychology and, 33
  Purkinje's description of, 107–109
  vivid, 70, 71
indirect vision, 11–13, 34, 42
individual differences, 36, 113
inflow theory, 61
inner ear, 16, 21
inner eye, 76
inner light, 44, 81, 89, 91
inner oscillation, 76
inner stimulus, 108
inner visual space, 82
Integrative Action of the Nervous System, 114
intellect, 36
intellectual faculties, 22
intended movement, 108
intended sensation, 108
interacting forces, 76
interference fringes, 56, 124
intermittent stimulation, 43, 53
interocular effects, 47, 122
interocular transfer, 52, 122
intrinsic light, 47
introspection, xii, 26, 27, 33
involuntary eye movements, 60
ipecac, 37
ipecacuanha, 26
iris, 9
iron filings, 104
irritability, 4
Italian, 30

J

J. E. Purkinje and Psychology, 37
jargon, 119

K

kaleidophone, 115
kaleidoscope, 106
keratoconus, 112
Koran, 113

L

labyrinth, 15, 21
Latin, 29, 30, 35
law, 30
law of nature, 67
lens, 5, 9, 10, 44
  and accommodation, 6, 7, 113
  artificial, 8
  as receptive organ, 10
  concave, 10
  convex, 10
  crystalline, 76, 77, 94, 97, 99, 100, 112
  curvature of, 5, 6, 113
  focus of, 91
  muscular activity in, 6, 7
lesion studies, Flourens', 23, 116–118
Leyden jars, 46
Libochovice, 29, 31
life phenomena, 33
light adaptation, 47, 48
light, 2–4, 79
  chaos, 47
  contrast, 47
  in dark field, Purkinje's description of, 81–82
  laws of, 88
  nature of, 3
  organ, 88
  perception, 87
  physics of, 2–4
  principle, 89
  pulses, 43
  sensitivity, 86
  white, 2, 4, 92
light and shade figures, 42, 43, 66, 87
  illustrations of, 69
  primary and secondary forms, 69–71
  Purkinje's description of, 68–71
lightning, 53, 102
Literary Archives of the Museum of Czech Literature, 35
Litomysl, 30, 31
long-sightedness, 5, 10, 11
luminous rings (*see also* firey rings), 67
  diagram of, 100
  Purkinje's description of, 100–102
Lunar Society, 18

M

madness, 108
magic disk, 43
magnetism, 108
magnification, 8
mammals, 22
maniacs, 18
maps, 125
marrow, 25, 87
masks for strabismus, 10
materia medica, 32
material realm, 88, 89
mathematics, 33
mean gray, 47
mechanical anodyne, 18
media of the eye, 87
medical art, 114
medicine, 30, 116
Memoirs of the American Philosophical Society, 34
memory, 108
  images, 62, 124
  training, 107
  visual, 67
mental activity, 107, 108
mental faculties, 33
mental illness, 103
mental image, 107
mental life, 36
mental phenomena, 36, 115, 124
metaphysicians, 115
meteors, 82, 97
microanatomy, 113, 114
microscope, 8, 25, 38, 54, 111
  achromatic, 2, 24, 35, 113
  Plössl, 24, 35
  simple, 113
microscopic morphology, 33
microtome, 24
Mikulov, 29, 30
mill-stone, 18
mind, 68, 107, 119
mineralogy, 31
mirror, 95
moiré fringes, 56
monastery, 33
  at Litomysl, 31
  at Olomouc, 30
Moravia, 29, 30
morphology, 33
motion adaptation, 15
motion aftereffect, 5, 56
  eye movements and, 14, 15
  interocular transfer of, 122
  neuroscience and, 24
  Purkinje's descriptions of, 14, 15
  vertigo and, 14, 15
motions of the retina, 20
motor control, 22
motor coordination, 22
mouches volantes, 57, 123
Mount Olympus, 33
movement detection, 12
muscae volitantes, 57
muscular action, 5, 6
muscular contraction, 46, 114
muscular misalignment, 11
music, 29, 33, 106
myopia, 10, 47, 77
mythology, 33

N

Nachbild, 51, 62, 124
narcosis, 104
narcotics, 17, 74, 76, 107, 113
natural colors, 52, 53
natural environment, 4
natural phenomena, 76, 119
natural philosophers, 115
natural sciences, 30, 31, 38, 68
natural scientist, 1, 67, 88
natural selection, 117
natural world, laws of, 88
nature, 36, 68, 106, 108
Naturphilosophie, 26, 30, 31, 115
nausea, 16, 37, 86
near and far vision, 42, 100
near point of vision, 6, 7, 10, 34
nearsightedness, 5, 8, 10, 11, 104
nebulous stripes, 80
nerve, 23, 26
  cells, 25, 114
  core, 86
  fibers, 24, 114
  mass, 88
  pathways, 111
  pulp, 114
  structures, 111
  substance, 85
  transmission, 46, 114
nervous diseases, 88

nervous humors, 17
nervous system, 22, 23
  anatomy of, 23
  communication in, 23
  functions of, 62, 114
  laws of, 114
  network, 26
  weakening of, 74
nervousness, 107
Neue Beiträge zur Kenntniss des Sehens in subjectiver Hinsicht, 34
neural marrow, 77
neural processes, 23
neurology, xii
neuron doctrine, 2, 24, 114
neurons, 23, 26
neuropharmacology, 26
neurophysiology, 15
  origin of, 46
neuroscience, 4, 23–26, 111, 114–116
  anticipation of, xi
  conceptual foundations of, 2
  dawn of, 1, 2
  definition of, 23
  origin of, 114
  physiology and, 26
  visual, 15
neuroscientists, 114
New Contributions to the Knowledge of Vision in its Subjective Aspects, 7, 12–14, 17, 23, 34, 38, 42, 50, 55, 120, 122
Newton's color disk, 69, 92
Newton's physicalism, 2, 4
Newtonian optics, 4
noise, 80
nuclear membrane, 114
nucleolus, 114
nucleus, 24
nutmeg, 26
nystagmus, 19, 20–22, 61
  direction of, 20
  postrotary, 17, 19–21, 61, 118

O

object recognition, 10
objective and subjective phenomena, 68, 119
objective psychology, 35, 36
Observations and Experiments on the Physiology of the Senses, 4, 64–109
observations and experiments, 68, 116, 118, 119
Observations on the Senses, 119
ocular spectra, 21, 51, 117
ocular torsion, 17, 20
Olomouc, 30
On Fantastic Visual Appearances, 118
Opera Omnia, x, 23, 28, 34, 37, 40, 65
Opera Selecta, 37, 65, 111, 124
Ophthalmologischer Bibliothek, 84
ophthalmology, 31
ophthalmometer, 113
ophthalmoscope, 111
opium, 26
opponent processes, 27
optic axes, 48, 83, 84
optic chiasm, 59
optic disk, 48–50, 57, 58, 85, 124
optic music, 106
optic nerve, 57, 82–86, 100
  entry point of, 66, 78, 100, 105
  fibers in, 57
  insertion in the eye, 48
  location of, 86, 105
  optic disk and, 49, 74, 79
  pressure on, 45
  Purkinje's description, 82–86
optical aberration, 126
optical corrections, 9, 10
optical instruments, 8
opticians, 6
optics, 44, 67
optometer, 6
Orbis Pictus, 29
orbit, 46
orbital cavity, 102
organ of speech, 108
organ of vision, 86
organology, 62
ornaments, 106
otolith organs, 23
outflow theory, 61
overconvergence, 47

P

pain, 45, 105, 106
painters, 70
papillary lines, 111
parallel lines, 92–94, 104, 125
  as stimuli, 55, 67, 94
  in engravings, 122
  regular, 56, 93

parchment, 86
pathological conditions, 68
pathology, 16, 67, 88, 115
pattern disappearances, 42, 49, 84
pattern distortions, 42, 55–56, 121–125
patterned afterimage, 52
patterned wallpaper, 55
peaceful coexistence, 36
peacock, 101
pedagogical institutions, 31
pedagogy, 106
perceived movement, 43, 56
perception and physiology, 2, 111, 115
perceptual fading, 49, 126
perfect vision, 7, 106
perimeter, 12, 13
peripheral vision, 5, 12, 13, 49, 57
persisting images, 53, 62, 67, 124
  afterimages and, 107
  duration of, 54
  Purkinje's description of, 107–109
phantasm, 52
phantoms, 41, 67
pharmacologists, xi, 26
pharmacology, 116
phenomenological method, 2, 42
phenomenology, 42, 44, 123, 124
  Goethe's, 2, 4
philology, 30
Philosophical Observations on the Senses of Vision and Hearing, 58
Philosophy of Nature, 30
philosophy, 30, 31, 116
  Faculty of, 31
  of sight, 2
  psychology and, 33
  Romantic, 4
phorolyt, 43, 44
phosphenes, 44, 45
phosphorescence, 73, 89
phosphorus, 81
photometry, 122
phrenology, 21, 62
physical and mental phenomena, 115
physical apparatus, 30
physical exertion, 97–99
physical laws, 71
physical realm, 88
physical science, 111
physicalism, 4
physicist, 88
physics, 51, 108, 115, 119
  of light, 2, 4
  Purkinje's study of, 30, 31, 33
physiognomy, 106
Physiological Examination of the Organ of Vision, 34
physiological laboratory, 35
physiological optics, 126
physiological psychology, 26, 27, 35
physiological sciences, 33
physiologist, xi, 67, 115
Physiology as an Empirical Science, 33
physiology, 31, 42, 68, 114
  afterimages and, 51
  experience and, 4, 24
  grammar of, 68
  neuroscience and, 26
  of hearing, 75
  of posture and balance, 16
  of vision, 58, 119
  pathology and, 116
  psychology and, xii, 26, 27, 35
piano forte, 54
Piarist order, 30, 31
pigeons, 22, 23
plant extract, 7
poetry, 2, 30, 36, 39
polarity, change of, 79
porcelain, 86
Porterfield's *Treatise*, 60
portraits, xii, 14
postrotary
  eye movements, 17, 19–21, 61, 126
  nystagmus, 17, 19–21, 61, 118
  vertigo, 14–23, 116–119
  visual motion, 19, 20, 117
postural control, 17
posture, 16, 21, 22, 117
Prague, xii, 29, 35, 36, 114
presbyopes, 57, 123
presbyopia, 9, 10, 77, 81, 82
pressure blindness, 45, 122
pressure figures, 34, 42, 44–47, 66, 121
  afterimages and, 88
  checkered appearance of, 45
  firey rings and, 58
  galvanic light figures and, 79
  history of, 44–46, 122
  illustrations of, 72
  Purkinje's description of, 71–77

scintillations and, 47, 82
secondary pattern, 73, 77
primary images, 104
primary sense activity, 108
prism, 47
private practice, 18
projection, 107
prolonged fixation, 55
Proteus, 33
protoplasm, 112
Prussian travel fellowship, 32
psychological data, 36
psychological experiments, 36
psychological faculties, 111
Psychological Fragments, 37
psychological speculations, 21
Psychologists in Word and Image, xii
psychology, 33, 34, 51
physiology and, xii, 26, 27, 35
of perception, 4
of vision, 15
Psychology of Vision, 65
psychopharmacology, 116
Ptolemy's board, 58
pulsating figure, 67
diagram of, 99
Purkinje's description of, 99–100
pulse, 99
pupil, 12, 37, 48, 104
accommodation and, 5, 56
aperture, 8
contraction, 7
diameter, 6
dilation, 7, 48
size, 56, 57, 95
voluntary movement of, 67, 95
pupillomotor response, 37
pupils, distance between, 83, 102
pure color, 113
pure science, 67
Purkinje
academic career, 2, 30–32
afterimage, 52
as medical student, 1, 2, 26, 31, 32
books studied by, 4, 119
chair of physiology, 36
doctoral dissertation by, xi, 4, 5, 31, 32, 37, 41, 111, 118–120
eyesight of, 9, 11, 47, 56, 58, 69, 71, 80–82
forgotten biological works, 39
Goethe's influence on, 2, 42, 121
inaugural lecture, 5, 12, 34, 37, 111
influence of Fichte's philosophy, 30
law of vertigo, 21
lecture notes of, 26, 27, 35
Piarist name, 31
portrait of, x, 27, 28, 39, 40, 63, 110, 127
psychological fragments by, 26, 27, 33, 35
reviews of literature by, 39
views of physiology, 26, 27, 115, 116
views of science, 27, 115, 116
Purkinje cells, xi, 1, 2, 25, 113
diagram of, 25
Purkinje fibers, xi, 1, 2, 113
Purkinje images, xii, 1, 5, 112
diagram of, 9
Purkinje shift, xii, 1, 5, 13–14, 113
color blending and, 42
description of, 13, 14, 34
Klotz's account, 14
Purkinje tree, xii, 1, 50, 51, 122–124
diagram of, 88
methods of observing, 51, 119
Purkinje's description of, 87–88
Purkinje-Sanson images, 113
Purkyně, xii, 124
purpose, 109
pursuit movements, 104

R

radiating lines, 55, 125
ray figure, 55, 56, 70
ray patterns, 42
real and apparent movement, 34, 42
real movement, 17, 108, 124
reality, 67
receptive organ, 48
receptors, 1, 124
reciprocal action, 52, 61
reflections from surfaces of eye, 5, 8, 9, 112, 113
reflexes, 23
refractive index, 113
regular geometric figures, 56, 106
reptiles, 22
reticularists, 25
retina, 77, 85–87, 89
afterimages and, 52, 107
as receptive surface, 50, 122
center of sensitivity, 105
image formation on, 48

retina (*cont.*)
location of phenomena in, 107, 108
microscopic structure of, 76
motion over, 15
peripheral, 113
persisting images and, 107
pressure figures and, 45
receptors in, 1
turbidity of, 87
retinal adaptation, 53
retinal anoxia, 122
retinal blood vessels (*see also* Purkinje tree), 42, 57, 58
diagram of, 88
Pequet's description of, 123
shadows, 1, 123, 124
visibility of, 50, 119, 121, 122
retinal circulation, visibility of, 57, 96
retinal correspondence, 59
retinal disparity, 59
retinal eccentricity, 60
retinal excitation, 91
retinal function, 45
retinal image, 3, 60
retinal images, combination of, 3
retinal structure, 51, 124
revolving stool, 22
rhombus pattern, 71, 73, 74, 92, 122
rods, 1
Romantic philosophers, 4
romantic physiology, 27, 62, 116
rose petals, 69
rotating bed, 18
rotating chair, 17, 18, 23
rotating flame, 53, 54, 92
rotating patterns, 15, 70
rotating sectored disk, 121
rotative couch, 18
roundabout, 17
Royal Society, 117
rubbish, 67
running, 99
Russian, 35

S

sand, 75
scanning, 60
Schlesischen Gesellschaft für vaterländische Kultur, 38
sciences, system of, 67
scientific recognition, 117
scintillating colors, 101
scintillating light patterns, 55, 66, 94, 125
intrinsic light and, 47
Purkinje's description of, 82
sclera, 100
seat of vision, 124
secondary images, 104
secondary sense activity, 108
self-administered drugs, xi, 26, 32, 113, 116
self-consciousness, 67
self-exploration, 116
self-knowledge, 36
semicircular canals, 16, 22, 23, 116, 118
sensations, 41, 49, 67, 68
sense, 36, 38, 109
external, xii
individuality of, 103
inner, xii
limitations of, 68
measurement of, 3
of vision, 86
specificity of, 68
survey of, 4, 39
synthesizing activity of, 70
topology of, 36
sensitivity, 4, 76
sensory organs, 67, 88, 107, 108
sensory phenomena, 68
sensory physiology, 4, 42
sensory realm, 68
sensory representation, 108
septum, 47, 59
sexual responsiveness, 22
shadow figures, 42
shimmer, 80
shooting stars, 53, 97
short sightedness, 5, 8, 10, 11, 104
sickness, 4
sight, 4, 68
philosophy of, 2, 4
singing, 29
single vision, 42, 58, 59, 122
Purkinje's description of, 102–104
theory of, 59
size perception, 120
sleep, 34, 104, 105, 109
as treatment, 18
neural nature of, 112
Purkinje's writing on, 36, 38
smell, 26
smelling salts, 77

Smith's *Optik*, 84
Smith's *Remarks*, 49
Society of German natural scientists, 37
soliloquy, 108
somatosensory aftereffects, 17
soul, 109
sounding body, 75
space, 62
  experience of, 117
  perception, 5, 35
  time and, 3, 115
spatial experience, 117
spatial frequency, 124
spatial oscillation, 76
spatial relations, 103
spatial vision, 3
specific nerve energies, 122
spectra, 19–21, 57
spectral sensitivity, 1
speculation, 20
speculum, 50
speech, 108
spider web figures, 34
spinal cord, 114
spiral of rectangles, 70, 73
spirals, 42, 106
squinting (*see also* strabismus), 11, 34, 42, 83
stabilized retinal image, 51, 61, 126
staining cells, 25
star pattern, 67, 98
star, 7
Stara Voda (Old Water), 30
steady fixation, 55, 126
Steinbuch's theory of vision, 5
stereometric images, 107, 122
stereopsis, 11, 122
stereoscope, 3, 58, 115, 119
stereoscopic depth perception, 58, 59, 122
stimulating colors, 69
stooping, 16
strabismus, 5, 10–11
stramonium, 26
Straznice, 30
stroboscope, 3, 42
stroboscopic disk, 43
stroboscopic patterns, 42–44, 49, 121
structure and function, 114
subjective colors, 121, 125
subjective experience, 1, 116, 126
  objective correlates of, 4, 88
subjective psychology, 36
subjective realm, 88
subjective sensations, 126
subjective sensory phenomena, 41, 67
subjective vision, 115, 119, 121, 124
subjective visual phenomena, 38
  history of, 41–62
  Müller's book, 115, 118
  Purkinje's descriptions of, 66–109
substantia albuginea, 9
successive motion contrast, 15
Sun, 52, 69, 91
sunlight, 70, 81, 113
sunrise, 1
superficial vision, 106
suppression, 11
swinging, 18
Symbolae ad ovi avium, 37
symmetry, 106
synapse, 26, 115

T

tactile space, 83
taste, 26
telescope, 8, 54
temperature, 108
theology, 30
Theory of colors, 2
theory of vison, 100
therapy, 46, 77, 116
thermometer, 6, 7
thresholds for detecting body rotation, 22
tone, 75, 76, 79
touch, 21, 103, 106
training, 107
transcendental aesthetics, 3
translation, 65, 118, 119
tree rings, 69, 77
trichromatic theory of color, 2
Troxler effect, 49
  Purkinje's description of, 84
turbidity in the eye, 50
turning the eye, 85, 96, 100
turpentine, 26
twilight, 88

U

Über die phantastischen Gesichtserscheinungen, 118
umbræ, 50

unconscious muscular actions, 17
uncoordinated movements, 117
units of measurement, 66
Universitas Carolo-Ferdinandea, 31
University of Breslau, 5, 34
University of Prague, 31, 36, 114
  Medical Faculty, 31
  Philosophical Faculty, 31
  Physiological Institute, 36
University of Vratislavia, 34

V

V5 (visual area 5), 124
vascular pattern of eye (*see also* Purkinje tree), 66, 73, 99–101
  Purkinje's description of, 87–88
vascular system, 16, 97
venesection, 18
verbal reports, 71, 77
vergence, 11
vertigo, 14–23, 60, 86, 116–119
  Darwin's speculations on, 4, 17–21, 62
  electrical stimulation and, 122
  eye movements and, 17, 19–21, 61, 126
  Flourens' experiments on, 116–118
  in the blind, 20
  introspective reports, 17
  motion aftereffects and, 14
  physiological significance of, 117
  Purkinje's experiments on, 5, 14–17, 21, 38, 39
  vestibular system and, 15, 16, 21–23
  Wells' experiments on, 17, 19–21, 117, 118
vestibular end-organs, 15
vestibular receptors, 22
vestibular system, 15, 16, 21–23, 116–118
veterinary science, 32
vibrating strings, 54
violin, 29
virtuosity, 106
vis nervosa, 114
visceral sensations, 20
visible spectrum, 3
vision
  as observational discipline, 3
  biology and, 1
  experimental discipline of, 3, 115
  individual differences in, 8, 9
  instruments for studying, 3, 115
  peripheral, 5, 12, 13, 49, 57
  physiological operation of, 109
  revolution in study of, 3, 4, 115
  theory of, 66, 115
  therapeutic investigations of, 8
visual acuity, 8, 11
visual aftereffects (*see also* motion aftereffect), 23
visual angle, 103
visual artists, 55
visual axes, 11, 49, 51, 59, 124
  convergence of, 104
  crossed, 103
  parallel, 104
visual direction, 58, 61
visual faculty, 59
visual field, 69, 70, 74, 77
  center of, 105
  elliptical, 78
  extent of, 11, 12
  fusion of, 81, 102, 103
  nasal, 12, 13
  of each eye, 101, 103
  outer limits of, 97, 100
  struggle between two, 81
  temporal, 12, 13
visual illusions, 2, 41
visual images, 106
visual memory, 67
  Purkinje's description of, 107–109
visual motion, 15
visual orientation, 117
visual persistence, 43, 51–54, 60
visual scientists, 55, 124
visual space, 36
visual spirit, 59
visual truths, 2
visual vertical, 23
visual vertigo, 62, 86, 116–119
  Dawin's analysis of, 17, 20
  history of, 19
  Purkinje's experiments on, xii, 38, 39, 60
visual-vestibular interaction, 21
vital processes, 116
vitreous body, 45, 76, 77, 98
volition, 4
voltaic current, 122

voltaic pile, 46, 77, 78
voluntary movement of the pupil, 95
voluntary squinting, 11

W

Wagner's *Handwörterbuch*, 36, 38
wakefulness, 36, 112
walking movements, 43
wandering cloudy stripes, xii, 66
  diagram of, 80
  Purkinje's description of, 79–81
waterfall illusion, 15
wavelength, 121
waves, 75, 76
waviness, 94, 95, 106
weeds, 67
weight, 108
whirling the body, 18
white matter, 24
will, 81, 95, 107, 108
windmill, 73
window, 91
winking, 52
winter, 74, 77
World in Pictures, 29

Y

yellow matter, 24
yellow spot, 51
Young's astigmatism, 50
Young's optometer, 6

Z

zigzag lines, 42, 69, 94
zigzag motion, 56
zigzag scintillations, 67, 94
  Purkinje's description of, 94
zinc pole, 46, 77, 78
zonule, 113
Zoonomia, 4, 17, 18, 20, 21, 118

For Product Safety Concerns and Information please contact our EU representative GPSR@taylorandfrancis.com
Taylor & Francis Verlag GmbH, Kaufingerstraße 24, 80331 München, Germany

www.ingramcontent.com/pod-product-compliance
Ingram Content Group UK Ltd.
Pitfield, Milton Keynes, MK11 3LW, UK
UKHW022120190926
475702UK00013B/1560

* 9 7 8 0 4 1 5 6 5 1 2 1 9 *